STUDENT WORKBOOK for

FIFTH EDITION

Anatomy of WRITING FOR PUBLICATION FOR NURSES

CYNTHIA SAVER, MS, RN

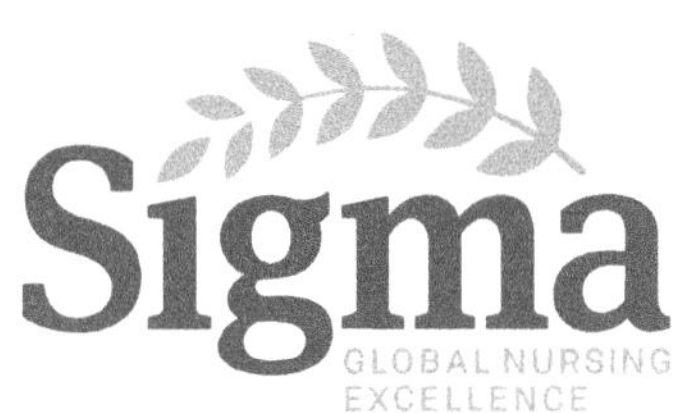

Sigma Theta Tau International Honor Society of Nursing (Sigma) is a nonprofit organization whose mission is advancing world health and celebrating nursing excellence in scholarship, leadership, and service. Founded in 1922, Sigma has more than 135,000 active members in over 100 countries and territories. Members include practicing nurses, instructors, researchers, policymakers, entrepreneurs, and others. Sigma's more than 540 chapters are located at more than 700 institutions of higher education throughout Armenia, Australia, Botswana, Brazil, Canada, Colombia, England, Eswatini, Ghana, Hong Kong, Ireland, Israel, Jamaica, Japan, Jordan, Kenya, Lebanon, Malawi, Mexico, the Netherlands, Nigeria, Pakistan, Philippines, Portugal, Puerto Rico, Scotland, Singapore, South Africa, South Korea, Sweden, Taiwan, Tanzania, Thailand, the United States, and Wales. Learn more at www.sigmanursing.org.

Sigma Theta Tau International
550 West North Street
Indianapolis, IN, USA 46202

To request a review copy for course adoption, order additional books, buy in bulk, or purchase for corporate use, contact Sigma Marketplace at 888.654.4968 (US/Canada toll-free) or +1.317.634.8171 (International), or solutions@sigmamarketplace.org.

To request author information, or for speaker or other media requests, contact Sigma Marketing at 888.634.7575 (US/Canada) or +1.317.634.8171 (International).

PRINT ISBN: 9781646481682
ISBN EPUB: 9781646481699
PDF ISBN: 9781646481750

Publisher: Dustin Sullivan
Managing Editor: Carla Hall
Acquisitions Editor: Emily Hatch
Publications Specialist: Todd Lothery
Development Editor: Jillmarie Leeper Sycamore
Project Editor: Jillmarie Leeper Sycamore
Cover Designer: Rebecca Batchelor
Copy Editor: Erin Geile
Interior Design/Page Layout: Kim Scott/Bumpy Design
Proofreader: Todd Lothery

To all my writing mentors over the years, my family (especially my mother, who introduced me to the pleasure of reading and writing), and Jackie, Terry, and David.

Acknowledgments

Thank you to my incredible team of contributors, most of whom have been with me through all five editions of this book. I am honored to be in such stellar company. The contributors bring a wonderful wealth of collective knowledge that reflects all the roles of publishing—author, editor, peer reviewer, designer, publisher—along with a strong commitment to help nurses share their expertise through publishing. I truly appreciate how they have generously shared their talents. I also appreciate the many others who read portions of the book and gave valuable feedback.

Thanks to Joan Borgatti for first linking anatomy to writing and to Patricia Dwyer Schull for her insightful comments and unfailing support.

Special thanks to the talented staff members at Sigma Theta Tau International, who always make authors look great: to Jill Sycamore and Erin Geile for their expert editing; Todd Lothery for proofreading; and Kim Scott for design and layout.

Publishing is truly a team effort!

About the Editor and Lead Author

Cynthia Saver, MS, RN, of CLS Development, is an award-winning author. She has more than five decades of experience in nursing, including more than four decades of publishing experience as a writer, editor, and senior vice president of editorial teams. Saver has written for many nursing publications, including *American Nurse Journal*, *American Journal of Nursing*, *AORN Journal*, *Journal of Nursing Regulation*, *Nurse Leader*, *Nursing Management*, *Nursing Spectrum*, *The Nurse Practitioner*, and *OR Manager*, to name a few. Her writing experience includes a 10-part writing for publication series for *AORN Journal*, research reports, case studies, interviews, clinical articles, and continuing education programs. She has written materials for nurses, physicians, pharmacists, social workers, physical therapists, occupational therapists, dentists, and other healthcare professionals.

Saver has worked with the top publishers as an author, editor, managing editor, and editorial director, including Editorial Director for *American Nurse Journal*, the official journal of the American Nurses Association, and Executive Vice President of Editorial for *Nursing Spectrum*. She was an invited reviewer for the *Publication Manual of the American Psychological Association* (7th ed., 2020). Saver's writing for publication program for nurses has received excellent reviews, and participants have published many articles. She received her master's degree in nursing from The Ohio State University, is an author-in-residence for *Nurse Author & Editor*, serves on the editorial board for *The Maryland Nurse*, and blogs for *American Nurse Journal* at The Writing Mind (https://www.myamericannurse.com/category/the-writing-mind).

About the Contributing Authors

Mary Alexander, MA, RN, CRNI, CAE, FAAN, is Chief Executive Officer Emerita at the Infusion Society (INS). She was named CEO of the INS and the Infusion Nurses Certification Corporation (INCC) in 1997 and served until her retirement in 2023. For 25 years as Editor of the *Journal of Infusion Nursing*, Alexander wrote bimonthly columns and had editorial responsibilities for *INSider*, the bimonthly membership newsletter. She is Editor of *Core Curriculum for Infusion Nursing* (5th ed.) and Editor-in-Chief of the INS textbook *Infusion Nursing: An Evidence-Based Approach*. Alexander's areas of expertise include infusion therapy with an emphasis on patient safety, practitioner competency, and standards development. Her clinical experience spans a variety of practice settings, including home care, alternative sites, and acute care settings.

Nancy J. Brent, JD, MS, RN, is a nurse attorney in private law practice. After practicing and teaching psychiatric nursing for more than 15 years, Brent graduated from Loyola University of Chicago School of Law in 1981. Her private practice is concentrated in professional licensure defense for nurses and other healthcare providers, consultation to nurses and school of nursing faculty, and educational programs in law and nursing practice for nurses and other healthcare groups. She has published extensively in the area of law and nursing practice. Brent is also the author of a legal blog at Nurse.com (https://www.nurse.com/blog/author/nbrent).

Christopher Burton, DPhil, RN, is Professor of Health Services Research, Health Foundation Improvement Science Fellow, Canterbury Christ Church University, Canterbury, Kent, England. Burton is a registered nurse with a special interest in supporting patients affected by stroke and long-term health conditions. As Professor of Health Services Research at Canterbury Christ Church University, he leads a programme of research and scholarship that seeks to close the gap between evidence, policy, and practice. He works with researchers across the globe to develop knowledge of "what works" in implementation and improvement and networks to embed this within educational programmes for nurses and other healthcare professionals.

Marianne Ditomassi, DNP, MBA, RN, NEA-BC, FAAN, is Executive Director of Nursing and Patient Care Services Operations and Magnet® Recognition at Massachusetts General Hospital (MGH). Ditomassi is the Chief of Staff for the Senior Vice President for Patient Care and Chief Nurse, who oversees the operations of nursing, therapy departments, and social services. Ditomassi's key areas of accountability include strategic planning, professional practice environment development and evaluation, recruitment and retention initiatives, business planning, fundraising, and communications. She also is the Magnet Program Director for MGH and coordinated MGH's initial Magnet designation journey in 2003 and subsequent Magnet redesignations in 2008, 2013, 2018, and 2023.

Susan Gennaro, PhD, RN, FAAN, is a Professor in the Connell School of Nursing at Boston College. She is an internationally renowned perinatal clinician and scholar whose research has improved healthcare for childbearing women and their families around the world. She is also the Editor of the *Journal of Nursing Scholarship*, which is read in more than 103 countries and whose mission is to advance knowledge to improve the health of the world's people. Gennaro has been active in supporting that mission by leading an understanding of how best to promote global dissemination of nursing scholarship.

Pamela J. Haylock, PhD, RN, FAAN, is a nurse educator and cancer survivorship consultant. Throughout her career, Haylock has held staff, advanced practice, management, nursing education, and consultation roles and is a past President of the Oncology Nursing Society. She contributes to professional and peer-reviewed literature as an author, editor, and manuscript reviewer, and by serving on professional journals' editorial boards. Her introduction to writing for general audiences was as coauthor of *Women's Cancers: How to Prevent Them, How to Treat Them, How to Beat Them* (with Kerry A. McGinn), followed by *Cancer Doesn't Have to Hurt* (with coauthor Carol P. Curtiss), and as editor and contributor for *Men's Cancers: How to Prevent Them, How to Treat Them, How to Beat Them.* Haylock was a team member and writer for the National Coalition for Cancer Survivorship's award-winning *Cancer Survival Toolbox*—audio instructional programs for survivors and family caregivers. In 2002, Haylock received the Distinguished Alumni Award for Service from the University of Iowa College of Nursing, and in 2008, she received a Distinguished Alumni Award for Service from the University of Iowa. She was inducted as a Fellow of the American Academy of Nursing in 2011.

Lisa Hopp, PhD, RN, FAAN, is Dean Emerita, Nursing, Purdue University Northwest; and Vice Dean, College of Nursing, Rosalind Franklin University of Medicine and Science, Chicago. She is internationally recognized for her work in evidence-based nursing practice. She has trained hundreds of faculty, advanced practice nurses, and library scientists in systematic review methodologies. Hopp is the founding director of the Indiana Center for Evidence Based Nursing, part of a global collaboration of JBI (formerly Joanna Briggs Institute) centers and groups that aim to improve healthcare outcomes through evidence-based healthcare. She continues to serve as a Deputy Director for a JBI Center of Excellence at Rosalind Franklin University of Medicine and

Science. She has been an educator for more than 30 years, helping prepare future advanced practice and registered nurses.

Timothy Landers, PhD, RN, APRN-CNP, CIC, FAAN, is a nurse practitioner and infection prevention researcher. His research focuses on practical, evidence-based infection prevention strategies to address the most pressing problems in infectious disease prevention. He has written multiple guidelines on infection prevention using a One Health paradigm. Landers was an Associate Professor at The Ohio State University for 10 years, where he taught in the graduate programs, and has served as the Nurse Scientist at Nationwide Children's Hospital. He was a Fulbright Scholar in Ethiopia from 2017 to 2018. Landers was on the editorial board of the *American Journal of Infection Control,* and his scholarly work has been widely featured in the media and lay press. He has mentored students and nurses in writing and publishing for many years.

Fidelindo Lim, DNP, CCRN, FAAN, is a Clinical Associate Professor in the NYU Rory Meyers College of Nursing at New York University. He has worked as a critical care nurse for 18 years, and concurrently, since 1996, as a nursing faculty member. Lim has published more than 200 articles on an array of topics, including clinical practice, geriatrics, nursing education, LGBTQ+ health, reflective practice, preceptorship, men in nursing, nursing humanities, and Florence Nightingale. *American Nurse Journal,* the official journal of the American Nurses Association, designated him as a Nurse Influencer. Lim is a Fellow of the American Academy of Nursing. He holds a DNP from Northeastern University, a master of arts in nursing education from NYU, and a BSN from Far Eastern University in Manila, Philippines.

Deborah Lindell, DNP, MSN, RN, CNE, ANEF, FAAN, is a Professor in the Frances Payne Bolton School of Nursing at Case Western Reserve University, Cleveland, Ohio. For over 30 years, Lindell has been an educator and administrator in undergraduate and graduate nursing programs. Currently, she coordinates Frances Payne Bolton School of Nursing's schoolwide Curriculum Transformation Initiative. Lindell's clinical background is in community/public health nursing, and her scholarship concerns nursing theory, history, and education. Internationally, she has consulted and taught masters' level courses in Vietnam and China and was a Fulbright Scholar in Kenya from 2021 to 2022. Lindell was instrumental in the development and implementation of the National League for Nursing's Certified Nurse Educator (CNE) Program and served as Chair of the CNE Commission. She is a Fellow in the NLN's Academy of Nursing Education and in the American Academy of Nursing.

Kayla Little, MSN, APRN, AGCNS-BC, PCCN, is a Clinical Nurse Specialist who supports the cardiovascular medicine, heart and lung transplant, and vascular surgery stepdown nursing units within the Heart, Vascular, and Thoracic Institute at the Cleveland Clinic Main Campus. She earned a BSN from Walsh University and an MSN from Kent State University. Little has been published in *Critical Care Nurse Journal, American Nurse Journal,* and *Clinical Nurse Specialist Journal.* She was an invited reviewer for the *AACN Procedure Manual for Progressive and Critical Care* (8th ed., 2023) and a contributor to *Foundations of Clinical Nurse Specialist Practice* (4th ed.). Little was the recipient of the Rising Star Clinical Nurse Specialist of the Year Award in 2022 from the National Association of Clinical Nurse Specialists. Her passion for mentoring nurses and future Clinical Nurse Specialists led her to be the recipient of the Barbara Donaho Distinguished Leadership in Learning Award from Kent State University in 2023. Little values lifelong learning and professional citizenship. She is a column editor for the *Clinical Nurse Specialist Journal* and serves on the board of directors for the National Association of Clinical Nurse Specialists.

Tina M. Marrelli, MSN, MA, RN, FAAN, is President of Marrelli and Associates Inc., a consulting and publishing firm. She is the author of 13 best-selling and award-winning healthcare books, including *Handbook of Home Health Standards: Quality, Documentation, and Reimbursement* (6th ed.); *Nurse Manager's Survival Guide* (4th ed.); *Hospice & Palliative Care Handbook* (4th ed.); *Home Health Aide: Guidelines for Care – Instructor Manual* (3rd ed.); and *A Guide for Caregiving: What's Next? Planning for Safety, Quality, and Compassionate Care for Your Loved One and Yourself.* Marrelli has also authored apps to assist with care planning. She received her BSN degree from Duke University and has master's degrees in health administration and in nursing. Marrelli has worked at CMS on Medicare home care and hospice Part A policy and operations, been the editor of three peer-reviewed publications, and practiced as a visiting nurse and manager in home care and hospice.

Cheryl L. Mee, MSN, MBA, RN, FAAN, leads the editorial team for *American Nurse Journal*, the official journal of the American Nurses Association. She is an Adjunct Instructor at Frances Payne Bolton School of Nursing, Case Western Reserve University, Cleveland, Ohio, working with doctor of nursing practice students. Her past roles include Editor-in-Chief for *Nursing* and Vice President of Nursing and Health Professions Journals at Elsevier. Mee has written over 130 articles addressing the current, persistent, challenging problems confronting nurses delivering direct patient care. She is on the board of Americans for Native Americans, where she has worked to provide scholarships, NCLEX fees, and varied clinical experiences for Native American nursing students, as well as planning annual health screening programs assessing hundreds of Navajo elementary school children.

Patricia Gonce Morton, PhD, RN, ACNP-BC, FAAN, is Dean Emeritus, University of Utah College of Nursing, where she served as Dean and Professor and held the Louis Peery Endowed Presidential Chair. Before her deanship, Morton served in various administrative positions at the University of Maryland School of Nursing. An educator and scholar who is known for her work in critical care nursing and nursing education, Morton has written multiple editions of three textbooks, numerous book chapters, and over 60 journal articles. She has served on the editorial board of eight nursing journals and for seven years was the Editor of the journal *AACN Clinical Issues: Advanced Practice in Acute and Critical Care*, sponsored by the American Association of Critical-Care Nurses. Currently, Morton is Editor of the *Journal of Professional Nursing*, sponsored by the American Association of Colleges of Nursing. She also is an author-in-residence for *Nurse Author & Editor.* In recognition of her contributions to nursing and healthcare, Morton was inducted as a Fellow in the American Academy of Nursing in 1999.

Cindy L. Munro, PhD, RN, ANP-BC, FAAN, FAANP, is Dean and Professor at the University of Miami School of Nursing and Health Studies in Coral Gables, Florida. She has served as Coeditor of *American Journal of Critical Care* for more than 10 years. An experienced peer reviewer, she has published more than 200 articles and presented at many national and international conferences. Munro received a diploma from York Hospital School of Nursing, a BSN from Millersville University of Pennsylvania, and an MSN from the University of Delaware. She earned her PhD in nursing and microbiology and immunology at Virginia Commonwealth University. Her NIH-funded research on oral care in critically ill adults has had an important effect on clinical practice. In 2016, Sigma Theta Tau International Honor Society of Nursing inducted Munro into its International Nurse Researcher Hall of Fame. She is an American Academy of Nursing Edge Runner.

Sandra M. Nettina, MSN, ANP-BC, is owner and founder of Prime Care House Calls in West Friendship, Maryland, and Editor of *The Lippincott Manual of Nursing Practice.* She attended the Sisters of Charity Hospital School of Nursing in Buffalo, New York; completed a bachelor's degree at Marymount College of Virginia; and received her MSN from the University of Pennsylvania, Philadelphia. As an adult nurse practitioner, Nettina's multidimensional career includes founding a nurse practitioner independent-house-calls practice; writing, editing, and reviewing for several publishing companies; providing leadership in her state nurse practitioner association; and volunteering for several health-related organizations.

Leslie H. Nicoll, PhD, MBA, RN, FAAN, is principal and owner of Maine Desk LLC and Editor-in-Chief of *CIN: Computers, Informatics, Nursing.* Nicoll has more than 43 years of experience in nursing and healthcare and has worked in clinical practice, research, and academia. She founded her own business, Maine Desk LLC, in 2001. Nicoll has been the Editor-in-Chief of *CIN: Computers, Informatics, Nursing* since 1995 and was the Editor-in-Chief of *Nurse Author & Editor* from 2014 to 2022. She served as Editor-in-Chief of *The Journal of Hospice and Palliative Nursing* for eight years (2001–2009). Nicoll is the author of more than 130 published professional articles, book chapters, and books, including *Writing in the Digital Age: Savvy Publishing for Healthcare Professionals,* coauthored with Peggy L. Chinn, and *The Editor's Handbook* (3rd ed.). She was the founding editor of *Perspectives on Nursing Theory.* In the non-nursing literature, she is the author of four "For Dummies" books, including *Kindle Paperwhite For Dummies.* Nicoll enjoys helping nurses and other healthcare professionals achieve their publication goals. She has done this through one-on-one support in her business as well as leading writing workshops for the National League for Nursing, a consortium of universities in Switzerland, and various colleges and schools of nursing in the United States. Nicoll became a Fellow in the American Academy of Nursing in 2014. She is active in INANE: The International Academy of Nursing Editors and received their leadership award for excellence in editorial publication in 2015.

Susanne J. Pavlovich-Danis, MSN, RN, APRN-C, CDCES, is Director of Clinical Continuing Education at TeamHealth Institute in Knoxville, Tennessee. She has 42 years of experience in nursing and healthcare in diverse clinical, academic, and consultant-based settings. As Director of Clinical Continuing Education at TeamHealth Institute, she currently oversees the Joint Accreditation for Interprofessional Continuing Education that includes the Accreditation Council for Continuing Medical Education (ACCME), the Accreditation Council for Pharmacy Education (ACPE), and the American Nurses Credentialing Center (ANCC). She serves in the chief editorial capacity for more than 600 annual continuing education activities nationwide for a multidisciplinary audience. She also maintains a private adult primary care practice in Plantation, Florida, and is a certified diabetes care and education specialist (CDCES). Pavlovich-Danis is an approved continuing nursing education provider for the Florida Board of Nursing. She has been published in the nursing literature more than 500 times since 1996 and lectured nationally and internationally.

Demetrius J. Porche, DNS, PhD, PCC, ANEF, FACHE, FAANP, FAAN, is Dean and Professor at the Louisiana State University Health Sciences Center School of Nursing in New Orleans. Porche is Chief Editor of the *American Journal of Men's Health* and was Associate Editor of the *Journal of the Association of Nurses in AIDS* for 10 years. He is a Virginia Henderson Fellow of Sigma Theta Tau International and a Society of Luther Christman Fellow for Contributions to Nursing by Men. He is also a Fellow in the National League for Nursing Nurse Educator Academy, the American

Academy of Nursing, and the American Academy of Nurse Practitioners. He is board-certified in healthcare by the American College of Healthcare Executives. Porche is author of *Health Policy: Application for Nurses and Other Health Care Professionals* (2nd ed.) and *Epidemiology for the Advanced Practice Nurse: A Population Health Approach*. He has published many articles in peer-reviewed journals.

Jo Rycroft-Malone, OBE, PhD, MSc, BSc (Hons), RN, is Distinguished Professor, Executive Dean of Health & Medicine at Lancaster University, England. She has a nursing background and is a health services researcher who studies the processes and outcomes of evidence-informed service delivery in different health service contexts across the globe. Rycroft-Malone is also the Director of the National Institute for Health Research (NIHR) Health Services & Delivery Research Programme, which funds research to generate evidence to improve the quality, accessibility, and organisation of health and care services in the United Kingdom. She was the inaugural Editor of *Worldviews on Evidence-Based Nursing*.

Nadine Salmon, MSN, RN, NPD-BC, IBCLC, is a Curriculum Designer in the Acute Vertical at Relias, a leading provider of online continuing education for healthcare, senior care, and disability professionals. Salmon obtained her BSN in South Africa more than 30 years ago and has worked as an RN in South Africa, England, and the United States in various settings, including labor and delivery, postpartum, home health, and adult surgical units. She has an MSN with an emphasis in leadership in healthcare systems from Grand Canyon University. Salmon has served as an appraiser for the American Nurses Credentialing Center, is certified in nursing professional development, and is an international board-certified lactation consultant. She has been involved in creating nursing continuing education content and certification review courses for more than 20 years, and enjoys collaborating with subject matter expert writers, instructional designers, and quality assurance and education technicians in developing continuing education courses for nurses, physicians, and allied health professionals.

Patricia Dwyer Schull, MSN, BS, is President of MedVantage Publishing LLC. She has more than 30 years' experience in medical and nursing publishing. She has published, written, and edited many nursing journals, books, websites, and other healthcare publications. Her company offers publishing solutions that support and educate healthcare professionals, including developing and launching the award-winning publications *Nursing Spectrum and McGraw Hill Nurses Drug Handbook*, *American Nurse Journal* (official journal of the American Nurses Association), and *Journal of Nursing Regulation* (official journal of the National Council of State Boards of Nursing). Previously, Schull held executive management positions with Reed Elsevier (Springhouse Corporation) and Wolters Kluwer (Lippincott, Williams & Wilkins), where she was responsible for leading editorial, sales, marketing, and new product development of nursing publications. Before entering the publishing industry, she practiced as a registered nurse in direct patient care, hospital management, and staff education.

Stephanie J. Schulte, MLIS, is Professor, Assistant Vice President, Health Sciences, and Director, Health Sciences Library at The Ohio State University. She is a library director and faculty health sciences librarian who specializes in teaching students, faculty, and staff advanced skills to support evidence-based practice and research endeavors. Her research work currently focuses on librarians who work directly with basic or life scientists. Schulte teaches within the medical school curriculum as well as the biomedical sciences undergraduate program at The Ohio State University and leads a team of research and education librarians serving five health sciences colleges and a large academic medical center. She has been active in university governance, the Medical Library Association, and the Midwest Chapter of the Medical Library Association.

Rose O. Sherman, EdD, RN, NEA-BC, FAAN, is Emeritus Professor, Christine E. Lynn College of Nursing at Florida Atlantic University, and a faculty member of the Marian K. Shaughnessy Nursing Leadership Academy at Case Western Reserve University. Before becoming a faculty member, Sherman was a nurse leader with the Department of Veterans Affairs for 25 years. She edits a popular leadership blog (www.emergingrnleader.com) and is Editor-in-Chief of *Nurse Leader*, the official journal of the American Organization for Nursing Leadership. Sherman has extensive experience with both podium and poster presentations at professional conferences. She has also served as an abstract reviewer for numerous professional conferences at the state and national levels. Sherman is a Gallup-certified strengths coach and author of the books *The Nurse Leader Coach: Become the Boss No One Wants to Leave, The Nuts and Bolts of Nursing Leadership: Your Toolkit for Success*, and *A Team Approach to Nursing Care Delivery: Tactics for Working Better Together.*

Lorraine Steefel, DNP, RN, CTN-A, is Director of LTS Writing/Mentoring & Editorial Services for RNs and students. She is a professional writer and writing consultant who has presented webinars and writing for publication workshops to nurses across the country. Her experience includes teaching academic writing to all levels of nursing students, especially mentoring DNP students who are writing their capstone project papers and turning them into published articles. Steefel has been widely published in peer-reviewed journals, nursing magazines, and on websites. She served as the American Nurses Association representative to the Centers for Disease Control and Prevention (CDC) Work Group to update the CDC website on ME/CFS (myalgic encephalomyelitis/chronic fatigue syndrome). Her book *What Nurses Know...Chronic Fatigue Syndrome* was published by Demos Publishers in New York. Steefel is a member of the Research Roadmap for ME/CFS for the National Institutes of Health, which is creating webinars about the illness to identify research priorities to move the field forward. Steefel is the Associate Editor for Peer Review for *Creative Nursing: A Journal of Values, Issues, Experience & Collaboration*, published by Sage, and an editorial board member of the *Journal of Nursing Practice, Applications and Reviews of Research* (JNPARR), the official journal of the Philippine Nurses Association of America. She is a mentor for the Thomas Edison State University School of Nursing online nursing program.

Table of Contents

Introduction to the Student Workbook

Writing well is not the result of luck or innate talent. Writing is a skill that you can learn. You learn writing in the same way you learn clinical skills such as suctioning and venipuncture—through practice. This workbook, a companion to *Anatomy of Writing for Publication for Nurses,* Fifth Edition, provides you with multiple practice opportunities. These opportunities will help you build excellent writing skills.

The workbook also gives you the opportunity to further explore writing for publication. You may wonder why, given life's demands, you need to think about writing for publication. One reason is that publishing can help advance your career. Having your name on publications makes you more attractive to employers seeking to hire and to conferences seeking speakers. On the job, publications can help you move up the professional development ladder and open doors to new opportunities.

But the most important reason to publish is why we became nurses in the first place: to benefit patients. The benefit may be direct (e.g., helping nurses apply knowledge about a particular disease state or sharing the results of your research study), or it can be indirect (e.g., by sharing innovative teaching strategies with other faculty members responsible for preparing nurses). Either way, in the end, patients benefit. That's why as nurses, we have a duty to disseminate.

How To Use This Workbook

The *Student Workbook for Anatomy of Writing for Publication for Nurses,* Fifth Edition, summarizes each chapter, followed by relevant learning activities. These are called Write Now! to convey the intent of immediate application. You should read the chapter before completing the activities (you may not be assigned all the items).

Like the book, this workbook is divided into two parts. Part I, "A Primer on Writing and Publishing," describes the basics of publishing, from generating a great idea and writing an article to revising your manuscript and sharing your work. This section is packed with information on how to bolster the chance that your manuscript will be accepted for publication. Part II, "Tips for Writing Different Types of Articles," is where you can apply what you learned in Part I. Each chapter takes you through writing a particular type of paper or article, including clinical articles, research reports, review articles, books, personal narratives, continuing education content, and writing for consumers. You can dip into the relevant chapter in Part II depending on your writing goals (or school assignment).

I and the contributing authors hope that you find the workbook helpful.

PART I

A Primer on Writing and Publishing

CHAPTER 1
Anatomy of Writing

Overview

Writing provides the opportunity for nurses to disseminate their knowledge, which is one of our professional responsibilities. It also can enhance your career path, increase your own knowledge, and advance the profession. But many nurses can be intimidated by writing. It may help to compare writing to anatomy, with each part related to an organ (see Figure 1.1).

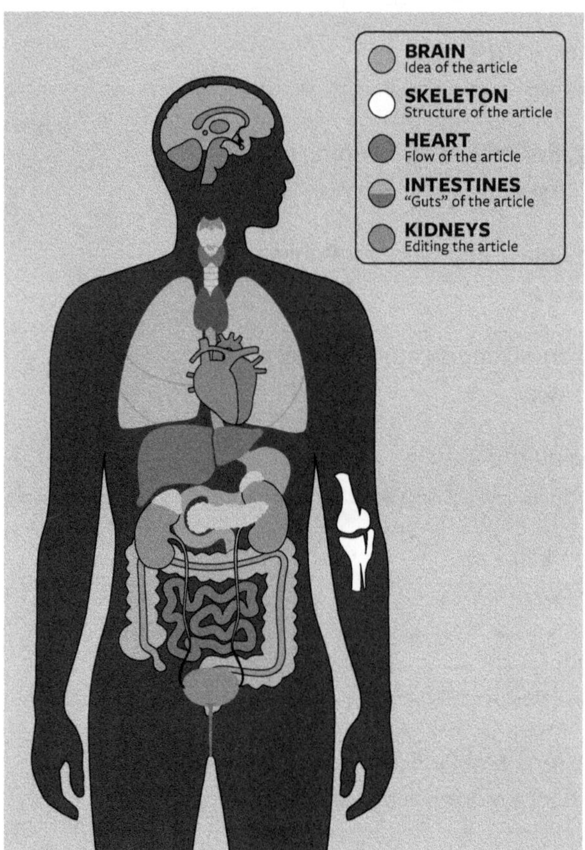

FIGURE 1.1 Think about writing in terms of parts of the body.

- *Idea* is the topic. Be sure it's not too broad for the planned length of your article. (In this workbook, "article" refers to the writing product, which can include anything from a blog post to a book chapter.)
- *Structure* is what holds the article together—a beginning, middle, and end. The beginning should entice the reader into the article, the middle should provide information related to the topic, and the conclusion should reiterate your main points. Structure options vary. A common structure for research articles is IMRAD—**I**ntroduction, **M**ethods, **R**esults, **a**nd **D**iscussion.

- *Flow* refers to how an article moves from one point to the next. One aspect of flow is how an article is organized. As with structure, organization options vary. For example, an article about keeping meetings more productive lends itself to "how to," while an article on a specific disease process might use the format of incidence, pathophysiology, assessment, diagnosis, treatment, and nursing care.
- *Guts* refers to what makes the article function and keeps the reader reading. You can use techniques such as examples, graphics, and case studies to hold interest.
- *Editing* involves dissecting the article to ensure that every word works to advance the topic and the text is grammatically correct.

Comparing writing to anatomy helps demystify it and reinforce that it's a skill you can learn. However, you likely will still face other barriers to writing for publication, such as lack of time. It's vital that you schedule time for writing and give that time the same respect you would any other important meeting. Manage your writing project like a work project, setting specific goals and a timeline.

When you first embark on your writing journey, you may want to collaborate with a more experienced author or be part of a writing team. (If you're writing for clinicians other than, or in addition to, nurses, it's a good idea to partner with clinicians in those specialties.) Like any team, writing teams can be effective—or not. Follow a few principles, such as setting expectations for participation, at the start to keep your project on track. Document the discussion for future reference.

Like nursing, publishing has a specific process to follow: submission, peer review, revision, editing and layout, author review and approval, and printed article. Understanding these steps will make the writing experience easier. You'll learn more about these as you move through subsequent chapters.

Write Now!

1. In the space below, list three benefits you feel will come from writing an article. It might be personal satisfaction, a desire to learn more about a topic, or something else. The point is that it should be personal to you.

   ____

   ____

   ____

2. Write a few sentences about how you will carve out time in your schedule to write. Create action steps—for example, when will you set your first writing date in your calendar?

   ____

   ____

   ____

3. Consider this scenario: You are on a writing team of four people. The final draft of the article is done, but one person repeatedly ignores requests for input. What would you do? How could this situation have been avoided?

4. Here is another scenario: You want to write an article on strategies for improving nutrition in hospitalized patients. Who would be good writing team members for this topic?

5. Use the editing checklist in the Additional Resources section for your next writing project.

CHAPTER 2
Finding, Refining, and Defining a Topic

Overview

Every good article starts with a good idea. Finding the right topic, and then refining and defining it, makes writing easier. Using this three-step process (find, refine, define) will help you develop your topic. In addition, you should rely on a journal's author guidelines to develop specifics for your article.

If you're struggling to *find* an idea, consider answering questions such as: What is happening at work or in my specialty? What can others learn from what I'm doing? Other questions can help you develop your idea more fully and identify the best place for publishing your completed article. These are reflected in the Write Now! section.

To *refine* your topic, focus it. A mind map can be helpful at this stage (see Figure 2.1).

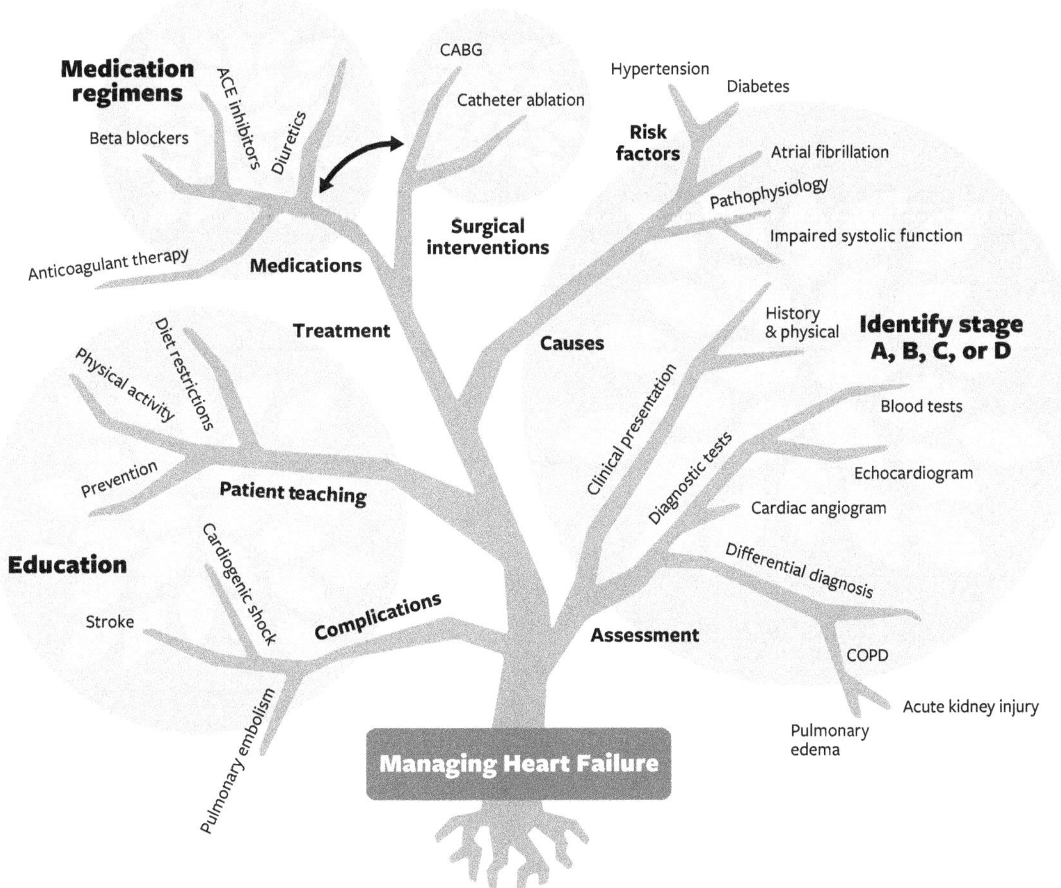

FIGURE 2.1 A mind map can help you visually analyze your topic and shed new light on how you might focus it.

When you feel you have sufficiently narrowed the topic, write a summary statement that sums up the article, including the target audience and purpose. Be as specific as possible. Here is a sample summary statement:

"This article provides staff nurses with an overview of three new antihypertensive drugs including pharmacokinetics, indications, dosage, adverse effects, contraindications, and patient education."

Subject your statement to the "So what?" test. Readers are busy people, so your article must resonate with them. Share your statement with others to gain feedback.

Once you have a summary statement, *define* your topic by determining the kind of article you will be writing (e.g., research study report, case study) and the type of publication you plan to target. When researching possible outlets, pay close attention to the author guidelines, which are essentially the policies and procedures for the publication. These guidelines include vital information such as types of articles accepted, the review process, and how to prepare and submit your manuscript.

Another step in defining your topic is to write an outline. Put your summary statement at the top, and then start listing main sections, with subsections under each one. Note any ideas for tables, figures, or illustrations. The outline will guide your writing process, shortening the time it takes to complete your writing project.

Write Now!

1. Use the right side of the table to answer the questions on the left.

Why should I write an article?	
Who will read my article?	
What interests me?	
What might interest others the most?	
What is happening at work or in my specialty?	
Which writing style should I use for a topic?	
What is the best timing for my article?	
Which publication is right for my article?	

2. Identify a topic of interest for your writing project. Use a mind map to narrow the focus of your idea. If you are stuck for a topic, consider how you would narrow the topic of "motivational interviewing." If you need more help with mind mapping, see https://www.mindtools.com/pages/article/newISS_01.htm.
3. Write a summary statement for your proposed article. Remember that this is one sentence that summarizes the entire article. Then see if it passes the "So what?" test by asking yourself why readers would care about the planned content. If you're not sure of a topic yet, write a summary statement for an article on pediatric delirium. Remember to be specific.
4. Create an outline for your topic idea.

CHAPTER 3
How to Select and Query a Publication

Overview

You have likely heard of the "rights of medication administration" (which, although not a complete guide for administering medications, is an easy way to remember key points); you can use the five rights below to choose the publication that best fits your topic:

- **Right audience:** Look for a publication that your target audience reads on a regular basis and that publishes the type of article you plan to write. Review the publication's mission statement, author guidelines, and several past issues.
- **Right access:** Access is a continuum, with completely *open access* (articles are freely available without a fee) at one end and *closed access* (a subscription is necessary to read articles) at the other end. Some research funders require works based on the funded project to be published in open access outlets. Check that the publication is listed in a reputable database such as the Directory of Nursing Journals (https://nursingeditors.com/journals-directory) or Cumulative Index to Nursing and Allied Health Literature (CINAHL). You want to avoid predatory journals that require unreasonable payment and low-quality journals.
- **Right timing:** Depending on the type of publication, editors may plan content several months ahead. Timing of events affect publication plans. For example, the COVID-19 pandemic disrupted many journal editors' publication plans as they worked to bring cutting-edge treatment information to their readers.
- **Right review process:** If you're planning to publish results of a study or quality improvement project, peer review will be particularly important.
- **Right metrics:** Metrics are used to determine the impact of a journal or article. Types of metrics are author metrics, traditional journal metrics, and journal- and article-level altmetrics. Some metrics have been criticized for a variety of reasons, so don't automatically dismiss a journal from consideration if it doesn't have a particular metric.

It's usually easier to start with a publication you regularly read, if possible.

Before sending off a completed manuscript, first email the editor to see if there is interest in your topic. Not all editors accept these "queries," but if they do, it's worth taking the step. You don't want to complete the manuscript only to learn that the editor isn't interested or already has an article on that topic ready to be published.

If the editor is interested in your topic, and you provided a deadline for submitting the manuscript, be sure to meet your commitment or, if you can't, notify the editor as soon as possible.

Write Now!

1. In the space below, list three journals you feel would be a good fit for the topic you identified in Chapter 2's exercise. Then rank them in the order of best fit. (If you're not sure of your topic yet, list three journals suitable for the topic of palliative care in patients with end-stage heart failure.)

   a. ______________________________

   b. ______________________________

   c. ______________________________

2. Evaluate at least one of your potential journals using the checklist from Think. Check. Submit. (http://thinkchecksubmit.org/journals).
3. Craft a query letter (email). You may find it helpful to use the template below as a guide.

Item to include	Your text
Name of editor, credentials, title	
Name of journal	
Brief statement of topic	
Why the topic would be of interest to the journal's readers	
Why you should be the one to write the article	
When you could submit the article	
Your name, credentials	
Your contact information (email and phone number)	

4. Consider this scenario: You are two weeks from the deadline for your article when you receive a new assignment and realize you won't be able to complete the article. What would you do?

CHAPTER 4
Finding and Documenting Sources

Overview

Authors need to find the best possible sources to use when writing their articles. This includes understanding what references are (and aren't) appropriate for a typical manuscript. For example, you want to use primary references (the original article or research report) whenever possible, rather than tertiary sources (such as encyclopedias). Secondary sources (e.g., textbooks or literature review articles) are those citations that quote the primary source document.

Components of a typical reference include:

- Author(s') names
- Title of article
- Title of journal
- Date of publication
- Volume
- Issue number
- Page numbers
- URL (Uniform Resource Locator)
- DOI (Digital Object Identifier)

It's important to format the references according to the style used by the journal. The two manuals that are most widely used in nursing and other healthcare publications are the *Publication Manual of the American Psychological Association* (7th ed.), published by the American Psychological Association, and the *AMA Manual of Style* (11th ed.), produced by the American Medical Association. These also have websites with subscription fees. The websites are updated between print editions as changes are made, so they are a valuable resource. (You may be able to access the websites through your organization's medical library.)

To find references to support your work, use databases such as MEDLINE (accessed via PubMed), CINAHL (Cumulative Index of Nursing and Allied Health Literature), and Google Scholar. In PubMed, you can enhance your search by using Medical Subject Headings—MeSH, developed by the National Library of Medicine.

Organizing references from the start of a project can reduce stress down the road by having all the necessary information in one spot. You might try a bibliography database manager (BDM) such as Mendeley. You can import articles into the BDM and then insert citations as you write your article. Most also allow you to change from one reference style to another. There is a learning curve for a BDM, but it can save you significant time in the long run.

Write Now!

1. Conduct a search for the same terms in PubMed and Google Scholar and compare your results. (If you don't know what to search for, try "moral distress in nurses.") Which returned more results? What was the quality of the results?
2. Here is citation information for a fictitious article. Format the citation as a reference at the end of the article, first using APA style and then using AMA style.

   Author: Latoya M. Smith

   Title: "Effectiveness of a Computer-Based App in Improving Adherence with Medications in Older Adults with Chronic Obstructive Pulmonary Disease"

   Journal: *Journal of Pulmonary Nurses*

   Year: 2024

   Volume: 14

   Issue: 5

   Page numbers: 13–22

   DOI number: https://doi.org/10.xxxx

   APA style:

   AMA style:
3. Download a free bibliography database manager such as Mendeley. Import some citations from the search you did in #1 into your library. Change the output style to APA, then AMA. Compare how the citations look.
4. Select three journals and identify the style of reference citation that each uses from looking at some articles. Then look at the information for authors for the journals. Do the guidelines specify which style manual to use for citations? Did you pick the right ones?
5. Watch the "PubMed: Overview" video at https://www.youtube.com/watch?v=1otz5qrUbxo, and then consider how PubMed and MEDLINE are different.
6. Improve your PubMed search skills by learning more about Medical Subject Headings (MeSH). The National Library of Medicine offers a free course at https://www.nlm.nih.gov/oet/ed/pubmed/mesh/index.html. For a quick overview, access the video "PubMed Subject Search: How It Works" at https://www.youtube.com/watch?v=6PhCRjQDfeI. For a more detailed video tutorial, access "How PubMed Works: Medical Subject Headings (MeSH)" at https://www.youtube.com/watch?v=xiHhFI_lG-U.

CHAPTER 5
Organizing the Article

Overview

The nature of the article you write will depend on the key messages you want to convey to readers, but the basic format typically includes a title and headings, beginning (introduction), middle (main portion of the article), and end (conclusion):

- **Title:** This tells your reader what the article is about. The nature of a title varies between formal and less formal publications, so review past articles for ideas. Titles for scholarly articles are typically longer and more descriptive than less formal articles, but for both, it's important to include keywords that will prompt the article to appear in the results box when someone searches the literature for a particular topic.
- **Headings:** These are "mini-titles" that break up the text in the main article and guide the reader through the article.
- **Beginning:** Craft an introduction that draws the reader into the article. Remember that the introduction sets the tone. You also want to reflect the style of the publication you are targeting.
- **Middle:** This is the main portion of your article. Use your outline when writing, and be sure that each paragraph relates to your topic.
- **End:** The conclusion should not introduce new information but rather reinforce key takeaways for the reader.

Many journals will also require you to submit an abstract. It's best to write the abstract last, after the main article. The abstract creates an important first impression for editors, peer reviewers, and readers, so give it the attention it deserves. (You may also need to provide keywords indicating the main topics of the article.)

Some journals are now encouraging authors to submit graphical (or visual) abstracts (GAs). These abstracts incorporate visuals that encourage reader engagement and help in disseminating information via social media. GAs may include icons, infographics, or flowcharts. Figure 5.1 is an example of a GA.

Be sure to identify a main message and keep the design simple. You can access free sample GA templates at https://www.simplifiedsciencepublishing.com/resources/best-graphical-abstract-examples-with-free-templates.

The type of article will partially dictate organization. Options include research (qualitative and quantitative), evidence-based practice, quality improvement, clinical, literature review, case study, and nursing narrative. Match the appropriate type to your topic and the publication you are targeting.

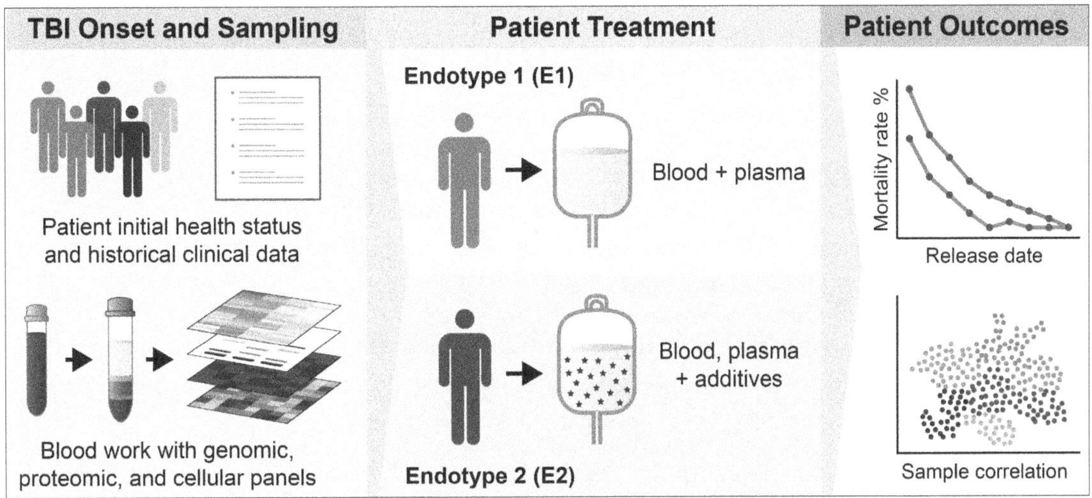

FIGURE 5.1 Elements of a graphical abstract. *(Source: Simplified Science Publishing, 2024. https://www.simplifiedsciencepublishing.com/resources/ best-graphical-abstract-examples-with-free-templates)*

Reporting guidelines are a useful resource for certain types of articles. These guidelines, typically developed with input from an expert panel, improve the consistency (and therefore usefulness) of published results. In fact, some journals require that authors use these guidelines (you can find that information in the author guidelines). Examples of reporting guidelines include:

- Standards for Reporting Qualitative Research (SRQR)
- Standards for QUality Improvement Reporting Excellence (SQUIRE 2.0)
- Preferred Reporting Items for Systematic reviews and Meta-Analyses (PRISMA)

You can find these guidelines and others at the EQUATOR Network's (Enhancing the QUAlity and Transparency Of health Research) website (https://www.equator-network.org). Reporting guidelines usually come with a checklist that can guide the organization of your article.

Write Now!

1. Choose three articles from two to three of your favorite nursing journals. List the name of the article and its type, such as research, evidence-based practice, quality improvement, clinical, literature review, or case study.
2. Pick a type of article you would like to write. Using a topic of your own choosing, summarize what you would include, using a template from the chapter.
3. Use the online tool from the EQUATOR Network (http://www.equator-network.org/toolkits/selecting-the-appropriate-reporting-guideline) to determine the most appropriate reporting guideline for a qualitative research report.
4. Compare the SQUIRE 2.0 (Standards for QUality Improvement Reporting Excellence) and the SRQR (Standards for Reporting Qualitative Research) guidelines. How are they similar and different?

CHAPTER 6
Writing Skills Lab

Overview

Basic writing skills are useful in all types of writing, from emails to journal articles to books. The four Cs of writing (clear, concise, correct, and compelling) can guide you in producing an effective manuscript:

- **Clear:** To enhance writing clarity, limit passive voice, choose effective words, provide signposts for the reader, and use parallel structure. Signposts include the use of transitional words and phrases such as "compared to" or "in contrast."
- **Concise:** Focus on what the reader *needs* to know as opposed to what is *nice* to know. That can be a challenge for authors with all levels of experience. Try to avoid long, convoluted sentences that are difficult for a reader to follow, and delete extraneous words (e.g., use "many" instead of "a large number of" and "may" instead of "could potentially"). You can use graphics and tables to be more concise and provide visual appeal.
- **Correct:** Proofing is an essential step before submitting an article. Check for accuracy of the text, including the references. Try to wait a day or two between finishing the article and proofing it so you can look at it with fresh eyes.
- **Compelling:** Help your article be compelling by taking ownership, being positive, and being considerate. Taking ownership may include using "I" or "we," depending on the style of the journal. It also means not couching major results from a study in weak terms such as "may be associated with" (unless your findings are weak). Being considerate includes anticipating what questions readers may have (and ensuring the answers are in the text) and using bias-free, patient-centered language.

Keep in mind that according to Schramm's formula, the amount people will read depends on two factors: what benefits they expect from the content and how much effort it takes to obtain the information. Therefore, a writer has two jobs: increase benefit and decrease effort.

Write Now!

1. Convert both of the following passive sentences into active sentences:

   Passive: Three main steps can be taken by nurses to improve pain management.

   Active: ____

   ____

   Passive: Phenomenological evidence of suffering and limitations wrought by pancreatic cancer that has been found in qualitative studies has resulted in an increased knowledge of living with pancreatic cancer.

   Active: ____

   ____

2. Rework the list below so that each entry is parallel in structure.

   To start an IV, the nurse should:

   - Wear gloves.
   - The tourniquet should be tied a few centimeters above the location.
   - The patient should make a fist.
   - Find an appropriate vein.
   - Cleanse the skin with alcohol.
   - The alcohol should be allowed to dry completely.

3. Identify the noun, verb, object, and qualifiers in the following sentences:

   The nurse finished her night shift on time.

   The trauma patient wakened to firm pressure.

4. Compare an article from *Nursing Research* to one from *American Nurse Journal*. How do they differ in tone, prevalence of passive/active voice, and use of references?

5. Pick an article from your favorite journal and identify active and passive sentences.

CHAPTER 7
All About Graphics

Overview

Eye-catching *graphics* (an inclusive term for tables, figures, graphs, illustrations, and photographs) call attention to key points in your manuscript. Study the target publication and the author guidelines to learn more about how graphics are used. The author guidelines will also tell you how graphics should be created and submitted.

Options for graphics include tables, line graphs, pie graphs, bar graphs, scatter plots, flowcharts, diagrams, photos, and videos. You can use the chart in Figure 7.1 to help you choose the most appropriate option based on what you want to convey.

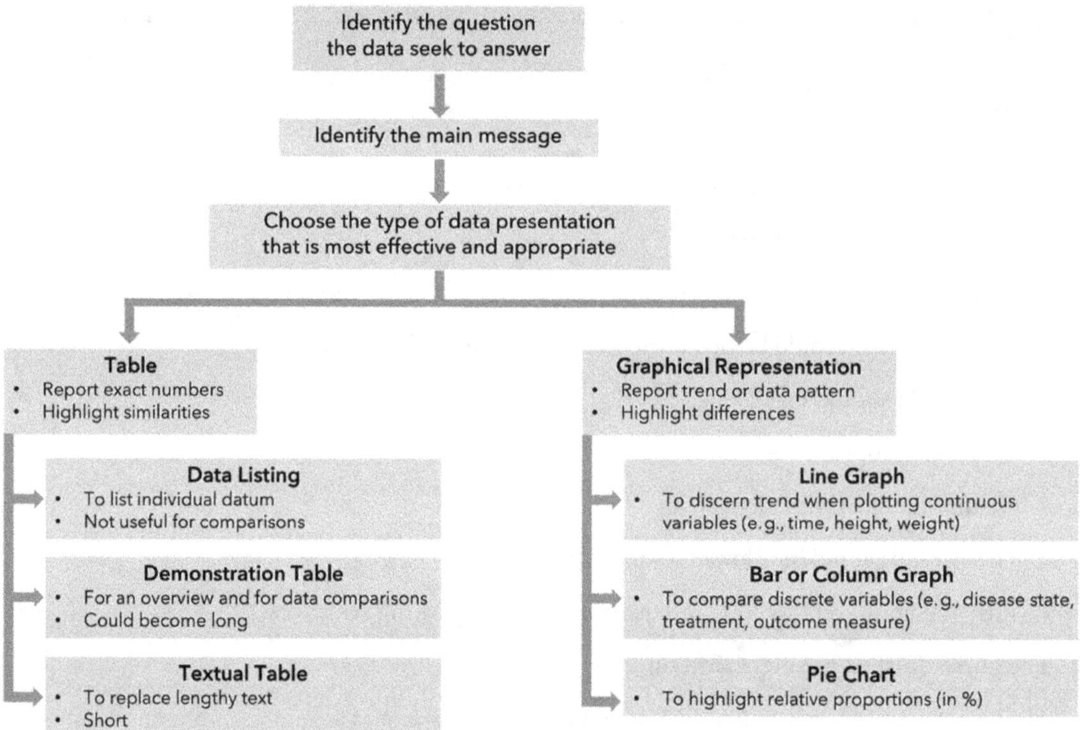

FIGURE 7.1 Algorithm for choosing how to present data.

You may also want to consider infographics, which combine text and images to deliver key messages.

Graphics should be clearly labeled and called out in the text whether directly (e.g., "The studies supporting the effectiveness of nursing telehealth visits are summarized in Table 1.") or in parentheses—for example, "Many studies support the use of nursing telehealth visits (Table 1)." Remember to obtain permission to use any previously published graphic, whether in print or online. To do so, you may have to submit your request via the Copyright Clearance Center.

Before submitting your article, you can use this checklist to ensure you have addressed the graphics aspect of your manuscript correctly:

- ☐ Are all figures and tables mentioned in the text?
- ☐ Are all figures and tables numbered in the order they are mentioned?
- ☐ Are all figures and tables numbered with Arabic numerals (1, 2, 3, and so on)?
- ☐ Do all tables and figures have titles?
- ☐ Does every table column have a heading?
- ☐ Are all tables and figures labeled using standard conventions?
- ☐ Is the font size acceptable for the publication (typically no smaller than 8 points and no larger than 14 points)?
- ☐ Are all data abbreviations spelled out in a descriptive legend (explanation key)?
- ☐ Are all figure elements large enough to remain legible if reduced to the width of the journal column or page?
- ☐ Is the figure resolution quality consistent with the publication guidelines?
- ☐ Have the figures and tables been saved in a format consistent with the publication guidelines?

Write Now!

1. Which type of graphic or table would work best for each of the items below (more than one may be correct)?

Purpose	Graphic
Demographics of comparison groups	
Certification among the sample size of critical care nurses	
Comparison of health habits of patients with and without heart failure	
Process of early assessment and administration of t-PA for stroke	
New type of ventilator	

2. Pick a research article and a clinical article to review. Analyze the effectiveness of the graphics in each. How are graphics used in each type of article?

3. In the space below, list three considerations for submitting an image to a journal.

   a. ______________________________

   b. ______________________________

   c. ______________________________

CHAPTER 8
Submissions and Revisions

Overview

Following the journal's author guidelines when you prepare and submit a manuscript will avoid an immediate rejection by the editor and helps set you up for success with peer reviews. Although the need to follow guidelines may seem obvious, many authors fail to take this simple step. The author guidelines typically include editorial mission, types of articles published, word count, editorial style (including which style guide is used), use of tables and figures, and how to submit the article.

Before you submit, do a final quality check of your manuscript, including proofing carefully. Submission is either through email or, more commonly, through an online editorial platform.

You'll also likely need to submit a cover letter that includes author information (including author order) and attests that the article has not been submitted elsewhere. You may be asked to state how each author contributed to the article and provide a conflict-of-interest form for each author.

In some cases, the editor may reject the article without peer review. If your article is sent for peer review, you will gain the benefit of experts reviewing your work to ensure it is high quality and will be helpful to the journal's readers. In most cases, this review is double-anonymous (also called double-blind), so the identity of authors and reviewers is not revealed.

After the review, editors commonly have three options. They may *accept* the manuscript, asking for only minor corrections or revisions. Acceptance at this stage is rare. They may ask you to *revise* the manuscript and resubmit it. Or they may *reject* the manuscript. Rejection after peer review doesn't mean failure. Perhaps your manuscript was rejected because reviewers had difficulty understanding the point of the manuscript, or too many questions were raised but not answered. Or you may have not chosen the best journal for your work.

Although the peer-review process is designed to improve the quality of what is published, it can be hard to read reviewers' comments. However, by making revisions based on those comments, you enhance the likelihood that your article will be accepted for publication. Unfortunately, too many authors abandon their article after reading the comments. Instead, take time to carefully read the feedback and revise the article as needed.

Before resubmitting your manuscript, convey how you addressed the reviewers' comments. A table, such as the one below, can help make this easier.

Requested Revision	Revision Made
Explain why you chose to use multiple regression (page 8, 3rd paragraph).	Added rationale for using this test (page 8, 4th paragraph).
Add a section on Jones's research to the background section (page 3, 3rd paragraph).	Section not added because of word count constraints and because Smith, whose study is already cited, found similar results in a more recent study.
Suggest moving signs and symptoms from text to a table (page 5, 2nd paragraph).	Created table (page 5).

After revision, hopefully your article will be accepted for publication. If so, you'll receive an edited copy to review before publication.

Write Now!

1. Identify a journal in which you are interested in publishing and review its submission guidelines and some past articles. Write a short paragraph with the key points you'll want to keep in mind when submitting an article.
2. The next time you have to write something, use the proofing checklist in the Additional Resources section of this workbook.
3. If you are a student, review the last paper you received comments on. Create a table that lists comments and your responses to those comments.

Comment	Response

CHAPTER 9
Writing a Peer Review

Overview

A well-done review provides objective, honest, constructive, and specific comments to authors and editors. You can become a better writer by serving as a peer reviewer. Learn more about writing a peer review by accessing resources such as:

- Enhancing the QUality and Transparency Of health Research (EQUATOR) Peer Reviewing Research Toolkit (https://www.equator-network.org/toolkits/peer-reviewing-research)
- Web of Science Academy Introduction to Peer Review (https://clarivate.com/web-of-science-academy)
- Sense about Science peer review workshops (https://senseaboutscience.org/activities/peer-review-the-nuts-and-bolts-2)
- Online tutorials from journals and publishers, such as those from Elsevier (https://researcheracademy.elsevier.com/navigating-peer-review/certified-peer-reviewer-course) and Wiley (https://authorservices.wiley.com/Reviewers/journal-reviewers/becoming-a-reviewer.html/peer-review-training.html).

The basic steps of a peer review include:

- **Complete an initial read:** This helps you gain an overall sense of the manuscript.
- **Critique each section:** It's best to leave the abstract for last. As you read, consider three categories of notes: positives, problems, and potential improvements.
- **Complete a final read:** Think about the manuscript overall. Does it provide new information? Would it be of interest to the journal's readers? Is it well organized? Then review the abstract again to see if it matches the content and review the title to assess if it is appropriate.

After these three steps, you're ready to write the review. Summarize positive aspects, and state any major identified problems (and whether it's possible for the author to correct them). Then summarize your comments in each section. It's important to be specific and, if possible, to provide concrete suggestions for addressing any issues. Include your thoughts as to whether the article should be accepted for publication, accepted pending revisions, revised and resubmitted, or rejected.

Be sure to keep any review you complete confidential, and never share a manuscript.

Write Now!

1. List three topic areas where you feel you would have enough knowledge to serve as a peer reviewer for a colleague's article.
2. Consider contacting the editor of a journal that includes your topic area to offer your services as a peer reviewer.

3. Access the peer review process at https://www.elsevier.com/reviewers/what-is-peer-review. Write a short description of each type of review:

Review Type	**Description**
Single anonymous	
Double anonymous	
Open	

4. Ask a colleague if they would be willing to share an article they have written so that you can practice your peer-review skills. (Another option is to pick a published article in a journal you regularly read.) After you review it, write a short synopsis of the manuscript and your overall opinion. Summarize the major positive aspects. State the most important problems you've identified, how serious you think they are, and whether it's possible for the author to fix them. It may be helpful to first make notes on your thoughts as you review the following areas:

Content	**Comments**
Introduction	
Body	
Conclusion	
Graphics and tables	
References	

CHAPTER 10

Publishing for Global Authors

Overview

Global authors make an important contribution to science, but they face unique challenges in selecting appropriate journals and in understanding ethical international standards. For example, language barriers are challenging for authors and journals alike. They not only prolong the time for dissemination but also incur costs for authors, who must obtain language assistance, and for editors, who must invest more time in the manuscript.

Tips for global authors include the following:

- **Fit your work to the journal's mission.** Be sure to review past issues of the journal and the author guidelines. You can submit to journals outside your country, but be sure your content will be applicable to the readers in that country.
- **If English is your second language, write in English from the start.** Although it's easier to first write in your native language, writing in English will help you be clearer and promote better flow of ideas. You may also want to consider translation and language editing services offered by publishers or publishing companies. Before choosing a service, conduct research to ensure the quality and ask about costs.
- **Use technology.** Some artificial intelligence (AI) tools that can help with grammar and some basic writing skills include Grammarly (https://www.grammarly.com) and Rytr.me (https://rytr.me). More advanced tools such as ChatGPT can help in organizing literature searches and preparing initial drafts of some sections of a manuscript (such as methods), but you must carefully check for accuracy. In addition, the tool doesn't verify the information it produces is original, so there is a risk of plagiarism. Any use of AI (other than basic spelling and grammar checks) must be disclosed when you submit the manuscript.
- **Collaborate with colleagues who are native English speakers.** These colleagues can help you develop an outline to guide your writing and review your manuscript before submission.

Global authors need to be aware of international standards for how scientific studies are reported, so that all the necessary information is included in the article.

Write Now!

1. Consider the challenges that authors for whom English is a second language face. If these authors cannot overcome these challenges, what will others lose as a result of not having access to their findings and insights?
2. Visit the *Journal of Nursing Scholarship* website and read one article from an author not from the United States. Summarize the article and its contribution to nursing.
3. The next time you have a project, consider involving an international partner to help you weigh global implications and possibly provide the opportunity to collaborate.

CHAPTER 11
Legal and Ethical Issues

Overview

It's important to adhere to ethical guidelines and follow legal requirements related to publishing. This includes maintaining patient confidentiality, respecting copyright, following guidelines when deciding authorship for an article, and not engaging in misconduct such as text recycling.

Just as you maintain patient confidentiality in your practice, you need to do the same when writing for publication; you also need to respect a patient's privacy. You can change identifying aspects, or, if you are reporting on a particular case study, you should obtain permission from the patient, even if you will not use their name.

Part of respecting copyright is obtaining permission to use previously published material (such as tables and figures) in your own work. In most cases, publishers either have an online form on their websites for requesting permission, or the website directs authors to the Copyright Clearance Center (https://marketplace.copyright.com/rs-ui-web/mp) to complete an online request (a free account is required).

Authorship should be determined at the start of a project, and only those who made substantial contributions to the article should be listed as authors. The International Committee of Medical Journal Editors (ICMJE) and a task force for the International Society for Medical Publication Professionals (ISMPP) have both developed authorship criteria. Most scholarly journals in the healthcare field use the ICMJE criteria. (Those who do not meet the criteria for authorship but contributed to the manuscript can be acknowledged instead of listed as an author.) All authors need to disclose any potential conflicts of interest, such as paid honoraria for speaking engagements for a company that manufactures a drug that is being written about.

Avoiding misconduct includes not engaging in text recycling. Text recycling can be appropriate, but it also can be unethical and illegal. The Text Recycling Research Project website (https://textrecycling.org) has many resources to help you understand the dangers of text recycling. (Note: Text recycling is becoming the preferred terminology, rather than plagiarism or duplicate publishing, which are imprecise.)

Write Now!

1. You would like to reproduce Figure 3.1, which shows a model of how to analyze delirium from the *Journal of Cognitive Dysfunction*. The model was on page 15 of an article written by T. Monk and G. Christie, which appeared in volume 6, issue 5, pages 14–20. You wish to use the model in your upcoming article in assessment of delirium in long-term care patients. Write a permission letter to the publisher (Publisher Group A) for the journal. (All journal information is fictitious.)
2. Visit the *Journal of Nursing Education* website at https://www.healio.com/nursing/journals/jne/submit-an-article and review its guidelines for submitting an article. Summarize the section related to human subjects protection.

3. Compare and contrast other requirements for publishing in nursing journals for consistency and differences.
4. Pretend you want to publish an article you wrote under a Creative Commons license. Use the Creative Commons Tool to find the recommended type of license based on your preferences: https://chooser-beta.creativecommons.org.
5. Your article has been accepted for publication by a nursing journal. The topic is one you wrote a student paper on, but the article is significantly different. Does the instructor who graded the paper and gave you feedback qualify for authorship? Why or why not?

CHAPTER 12
Promoting Your Work

Overview

It's not enough to simply publish your work. You have a responsibility to ensure wider dissemination. Start developing a dissemination plan as you write. For example, writing an effective title will help others discover your work more easily when conducting a search. Think about who would be interested in your work—not only other nurses, but those outside the profession, such as other healthcare professionals, caregivers, and the general public.

Ways to make your work more accessible include the following:

- **Plain language summary:** This is what its name implies: a summary of your work written in nontechnical language.
- **Graphical abstract:** This type of abstract uses images and short text to spark reader interest. It should include the background or setting for your work, methods, results or implications, author names and affiliations, and contact information.
- **Video abstract:** This is a short presentation of your work meant to engage potential readers. The video should be short and convey the key points. Speak enthusiastically and provide a call to action (what you want readers to do after watching the video).
- **Podcast:** Some journals offer the option for authors to be interviewed about their work by the editor.

Check the publication's author guidelines to see if it accepts or encourages these tools, which can be shared via websites and social media. Some publishers provide support for creating innovative visuals, although a fee may be involved. Many publishers also provide information about dissemination strategy.

Even if you don't develop these items, you should promote your work via social media. Provide additional content or commentary rather than simply posting a link. Give people a reason to react to your post and share it with others. Another avenue to consider is a scientific social networking site such as Research Gate (https://www.researchgate.net).

In addition to social media, you might want to write a guest blog. You also should create a professional profile on LinkedIn and register for an Open Researcher and Contributor ID (ORCID) and keep your profile current.

Here is a checklist to use when making dissemination plans for your work:

- ☐ Craft your title and abstract for search-engine optimization.
- ☐ Create at least one research profile on an academic social media site, and post your articles there, if copyright agreement permits.
- ☐ Post information about your published work on your own social media accounts. Keep the entries short and provide a link.

- ☐ Ask staff in the communications department of your organization if they will post the information on the organization's social media outlets.
- ☐ Add the publication to your curriculum vitae and to your research profiles (e.g., ORCID).
- ☐ Share the news about your publication with the nursing school you attended so it can be listed in newsletters and other publications.
- ☐ Network with others at conferences you attend, so you can share your work. It's also a great way to identify potential research collaborators.
- ☐ Present your own work at conferences.
- ☐ Be sure to include your contact information in slide presentations, handouts, and other materials, and add your latest article to the signature line of your email.
- ☐ Share your publication with two or three people who you think will be interested, and see if they are willing to promote it through their own social media outlets.

Following these strategies will help ensure your work reaches the most people it can benefit.

Write Now!

1. Identify two or three target audiences who might be interested in the topics you most like to write about, and then describe the top two points of interest for each group.
2. Pick an article from a journal, and then practice writing social media messages for X, Facebook, and Instagram that promote the article.
3. If you don't have one already, create a free LinkedIn profile. If you have started your research journey, create an Open Researcher and Contributor ID (ORCID) account.
4. Make a list of potential magazines or news outlets that would be interested in your topic.
5. Write a plain language summary of a review of your choosing. Aim to write it so that a person without any background in healthcare can understand it. What was the experience of translating what you learned from the review into a summary that a "lay" knowledge user can understand?

Part I Summary

Now that you have a sound understanding of the elements of publishing, you're ready to move on to Part II, which provides tips for writing different types of articles. The flowchart on the next page summarizes the publication steps.

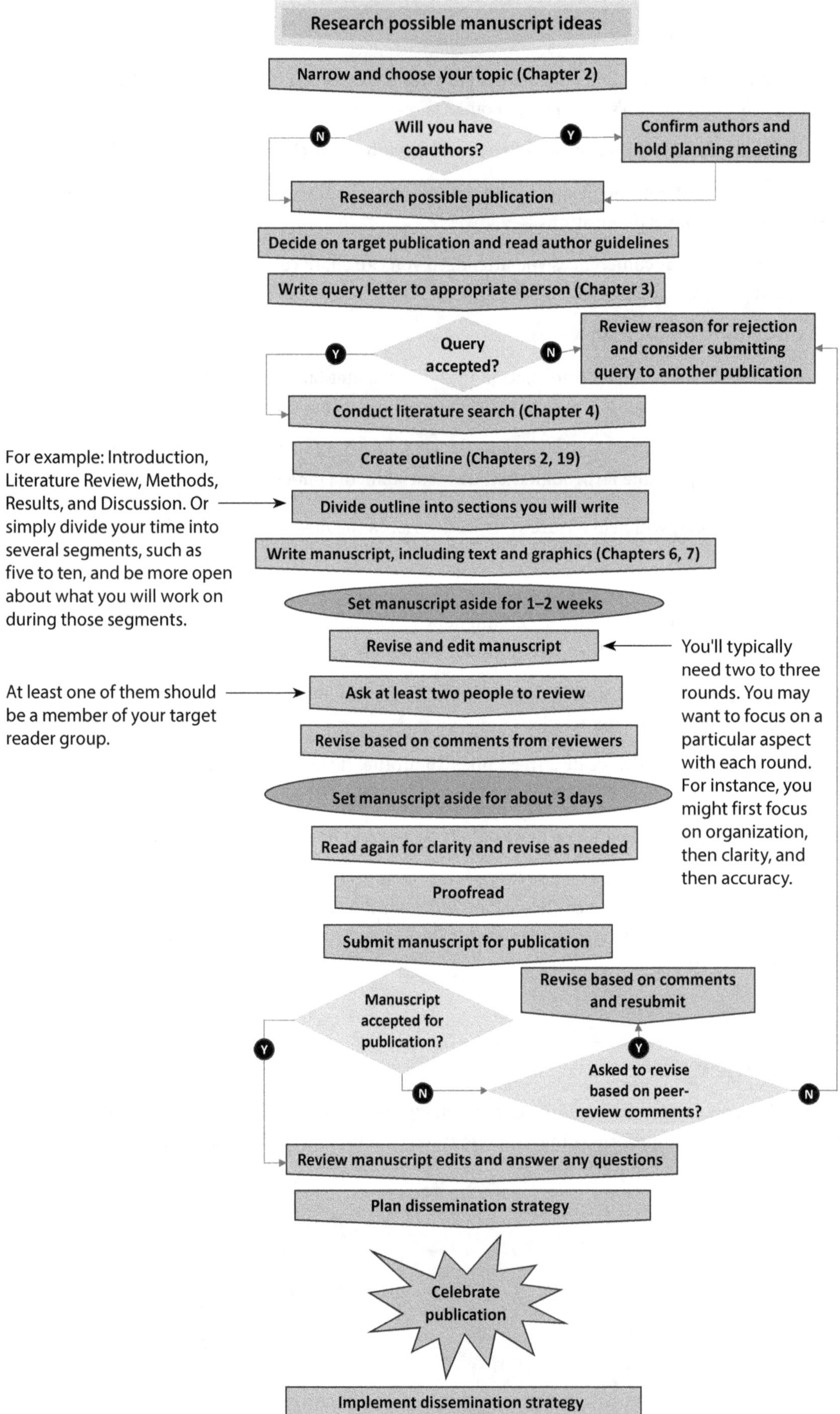
Research possible manuscript ideas
Narrow and choose your topic (Chapter 2)
Will you have coauthors?
N
Y
Confirm authors and hold planning meeting
Research possible publication
Decide on target publication and read author guidelines
Write query letter to appropriate person (Chapter 3)
Query accepted?
Y
N
Review reason for rejection and consider submitting query to another publication
Conduct literature search (Chapter 4)
Create outline (Chapters 2, 19)
For example: Introduction, Literature Review, Methods, Results, and Discussion. Or simply divide your time into several segments, such as five to ten, and be more open about what you will work on during those segments.
Divide outline into sections you will write
Write manuscript, including text and graphics (Chapters 6, 7)
Set manuscript aside for 1–2 weeks
Revise and edit manuscript
You'll typically need two to three rounds. You may want to focus on a particular aspect with each round. For instance, you might first focus on organization, then clarity, and then accuracy.
At least one of them should be a member of your target reader group.
Ask at least two people to review
Revise based on comments from reviewers
Set manuscript aside for about 3 days
Read again for clarity and revise as needed
Proofread
Submit manuscript for publication
Manuscript accepted for publication?
Y
N
Revise based on comments and resubmit
Y
Asked to revise based on peer-review comments?
N
Review manuscript edits and answer any questions
Plan dissemination strategy
Celebrate publication
Implement dissemination strategy

PART II

Tips for Writing Different Types of Articles

CHAPTER 13
Writing the Clinical Article

Overview

Because you're likely most familiar with clinical articles, they make a great starting point for you to start your professional writing endeavors. Clinical articles are read by all types of nurses and are published in many types of nursing journals.

A clinical article might include all or some of these elements: etiology, incidence, health disparities, pathophysiology, clinical presentation, differential diagnosis, diagnostics, treatment, and nursing implications.

The process of creating a clinical article follows what you learned in Part I:

- Develop a clinical topic and focus.
- Select a journal to target for submission.
- Send a query email to the journal.
- Choose an appropriate format.
- Gather information.
- Prepare to write
- Write using authoritative and active voice.
- Edit your manuscript.
- Submit.

Creating a timeline is essential; otherwise, your project will continually be pushed aside for other priorities.

Write Now!

1. List two possible ideas for a clinical article. Look for a prototype format(s) (e.g., case study, how to, disease state) that fits your topic.

____

____

____

2. Write a title for one of the topics. Be sure the title is enticing to readers. Also, try to improve on this title: "Compassion Fatigue."

____

____

____

3. Write a case study article on a topic of your choosing. If you are having trouble choosing a topic, consider this option: a patient who is newly diagnosed with diabetes.

____

____

____

4. Identify the subheads in the chapter or in a published clinical article.

____

____

____

5. Find the regular departments or columns in one or two clinical journals. Consider what topic you could write about that would fit one of them. (Review the author guidelines.)

____

____

____

CHAPTER 14
Writing the Research Report

Overview

A quantitative research report typically includes an abstract and then the introduction, literature review, methods, results, and discussion (IMRAD). A qualitative research report follows a similar pattern, as does a mixed-methods report, which uses both quantitative and qualitative methods. Here are the elements to include:

- **Title:** The title needs to be clear and accurate.
- **Abstract:** Provides a summary of the article. The content should be consistent with what is in the text.
- **Introduction:** This sets the stage for the report and explains why the study was important. When writing the introduction, you'll want to include answers to questions such as what is the problem, what is the problem's magnitude, who experiences the problem, and why was it important to conduct the study.
- **Literature review:** This puts your work in the context of past studies. It provides the reader with a synopsis of what is known about each variable in your study, what is not known, and how your study fills the gap. Either within or after the literature review, you may include a summary of the theoretical or conceptual framework that influenced the direction of the study. Right after the literature review, you'll want to include research questions or hypotheses.
- **Methods:** This section provides readers with a road map as to how you conducted the study. It usually includes these elements: design, sample, setting, procedures, ethics, instruments, and data analyses.
- **Results:** As the name indicates, this is where you present your findings. Provide key results in the text, and support them with tables and figures that provide more detail.
- **Discussion:** Here is where you interpret your results and explain their implications. Don't make the mistake of simply repeating the results.

You'll want to wrap up your article with a concise conclusion that recaps the main messages for readers.

Research articles need to be written clearly using accepted standards of research reporting so readers can evaluate the quality of the findings and their relevance for current clinical practice.

Write Now!

1. Read a published article without reviewing the abstract. Then use the OJISH mnemonic to write an abstract for the article and compare it to the published abstract. Use the table below to record your initial thoughts.

Step	Notes
Outline a pressing problem in the field.	
Justify a new study with a gap in the literature.	
Introduce the purpose of the proposed or present study.	
Summarize the methodology.	
Highlight the major findings.	

2. Review the abstract from the study by Zangaro and colleagues (2023) included in the chapter, and then formulate one or two research questions and several hypotheses you may wish to test if you were doing this study. Next, read the entire article and see if any of your questions/hypotheses match those of the authors.

3. Read the results section of two research articles and note how the authors have used tables and figures to supplement the article. Critique the two articles in how well they presented their results and the extent to which tables and figures helped you understand what the authors were trying to convey. What would you do differently?

4. Write the data analysis section for an article reporting the results of a qualitative study of nurses' reactions when caring for patients in the middle of a pandemic. Refer to the chapter for guidelines as to what you should include.

____

____

____

CHAPTER 15
Writing the Review Article

Overview

Review articles synthesize a large amount of information from previously published literature. The most common types in the nursing field are literature, systematic, scoping, and integrative. The components of a review article are similar to that of a research report:

- Abstract
- Background
- Objectives
- Methods
- Results
- Discussion

Table 15.1 is a summary of three key types of reviews.

Approach the review with a well-thought-out plan, so that it will be easier for you to write the results of what you have found.

TABLE 15.1 Comparing Review Key Features

	Systematic Review (quantitative)	**Systematic Review (qualitative)**	**Scoping Review**	**Integrative Review**
Methodological developers	Cochrane, JBI, and others	Cochrane, JBI, and others	JBI, funded researchers	Whittemore & Knafl,* with some development in the general literature
Typical aim	Effectiveness	Meaning	Map	Integrate
Clear objective and/or research question	PICO** or similar form	PICo or similar form	Broadly defined	Broadly defined
Predefined, published protocol	Yes	Yes	Yes	Not usually
Comprehensive, exhaustive, and transparent search	Yes	Yes	Yes, iterative	Iterative, less consistently defined
Dual, independent reviewers for retrieval and appraisal	Yes	Yes	Yes	Sometimes
Documentation of destiny of all retrieved articles	Yes	Yes	Yes	Sometimes
Data extraction tools represented	Yes	Yes	Yes, but iterative	Unclear
Appraisal represented	Yes, often in tabular form or represented as risk of bias	Yes, often in tabular form with appraisal of credibility	No; aim is to map	Unclear
Synthesis methods	Meta-analysis or narrative	Meta-aggregation or meta-ethnography	Summary rather than synthesis	Iterative and dependent on types of evidence
Ratings of evidence strength or certainty	Yes, usually GRADE methods related to certainty of findings	Yes, using standardized methods related to credibility and dependability of findings	No, although there may be a map of study designs found	Not described

Whittemore, R., & Knafl, K. (2005). The integrative review: Updated methodology. Journal of Advanced Nursing, *52(5), 546–553. http://dx.doi.org/10.1111/j.1365-2648.2005.03621.x*
***PICO = **P**opulation, **I**ntervention(s) or phenomenon of interest, **C**omparator(s) or **C**ontext, **O**utcomes*

Write Now!

1. Find an example of a systematic review, a scoping review, and an integrative review. Compare them carefully to differentiate their purposes, methods, findings, and conclusions.

2. Read a published systematic review without reading the abstract. Then, write one following the elements of a systematic review. Did you find similar conclusions as the investigators who published the review?

3. Find an appraisal tool for one type of review (e.g., find the CASP tool for systematic reviews). Read the review and identify its strengths and weakness.

4. Use the PICO (P = population, I = intervention, C = comparator, O = outcome) method to write a question for a systematic review.

CHAPTER 16

Reporting the Quality Improvement or Evidence-Based Practice Project

Overview

Although quality improvement (QI) and evidence-based practice (EBP) projects have distinguishing features, both are designed to improve patient care. They may be easier projects for a novice writer because reporting guidelines exist to help frame the manuscript. Examples of these guidelines include Standards for QUality Improvement Reporting Excellence (SQUIRE) 2.0 and Consolidated Standards for Reporting Qualitative Research (COREQ). You can find guidelines at the EQUATOR (Enhancing the QUAlity and Transparency Of health Research) Network website (https://www.equator-network.org).

Guidelines typically provide a checklist that can help you organize your article. The format usually includes title, abstract, introduction, methods, results, discussion, conclusion, and implications. When writing about what you did in the methods section, consider using words from a published taxonomy such as that from the Cochrane Effective Practice and Organisation of Care Review Group. This taxonomy includes four major types of interventions (see Table 16.1).

TABLE 16.1 Types of Implementation Interventions

Types of Interventions	Examples
Professional	Distribution of educational materials, local consensus processes, audit and feedback, reminders
Financial	Fee-for-service, incentives
Organizational	Revision of professional roles, skill mix change, patient involvement, changing documentation systems
Regulatory	Management of patient complaints, peer review

In both QI and EBP articles, it's important to provide details about what you did to help readers gain practical insights that might have relevance to their own work.

Write Now!

1. Think about a QI or EBP project that you have either led or been involved in. Write an outline for an article, including subheadings and sample text for each section. Consider how you might involve other relevant stakeholders in this planning process.

___

___

___

2. Pick a QI or EBP article from a journal and analyze it using the framework discussed in the chapter. How would you improve the article? The table below may be helpful.

____

____

____

Element	Your Comments
Title (Does it clearly convey what the article is about?)	
Abstract (Does it provide background, methods, findings, and conclusions?)	
Introduction (Does it explain why the project was done?)	
Methods (Does it clearly describe what was done, by whom, and where? Does it address ethical considerations?)	
Results (Does it describe what changes were made?)	
Discussion (Does it provide a useful overview?)	
Conclusion and implications (Does it consider implications and wider applicability?)	

3. Think about a QI project you have been involved in, and note what categories the interventions fell into using the table below as a guide.

____

____

____

Types of Interventions	**Examples**	**My Project**
Professional	Distribution of educational materials, local consensus processes, audit and feedback, reminders	
Financial	Fee-for-service, incentives	
Organizational	Revision of professional roles, skill mix change, patient involvement, changing documentation systems	
Regulatory	Management of patient complaints, peer review	

CHAPTER 17
Writing for Presentations

Overview

Following the guidelines in the call for abstracts improves the chance your submission to present at a conference will be accepted. The guidelines also can help you craft your podium and poster presentation so that it's most effective.

Be wary of predatory conferences. The work presented at these conferences is usually not peer-reviewed, and presenters are selected based on their willingness to pay registration fees and travel expenses. Consult with colleagues if you have any concerns, and use the checklist available at Think.Check.Attend. (https://thinkcheckattend.org), which suggests asking these questions before submitting an abstract:

- Are you aware of the society or the association organizing the conference?
- Have you or your colleagues attended this conference before?
- Is there clear information about the timeline and the agenda for the conference?
- Is the editorial committee listed on the website and, if so, have you heard of them?

Conferences can be low quality without being predatory, and these questions will help you identify those as well.

When writing your abstract, consider the audience so you can craft your content to appeal to them. Create an immediate impression with a compelling title that connects with the theme of the conference. Develop your submission in a word-processing document, and then copy and paste into the online form on the conference's website.

Your abstract will undergo review to see if it is a good fit and addition to the conference. If accepted, you will usually receive more guidelines that you can use to plan your podium or poster presentation.

Your *podium* presentation should be succinct and focus on key points. Keep slides simple and allow for about two to three minutes per slide. Practice alone and then in front of colleagues to hone your presentation.

Your *poster* should clearly present the key information. Your organization may have resources to help with design, or you can access online resources such as those from the University of North Carolina (https://gradschool.unc.edu/academics/resources/postertips.html). You can use Microsoft Word, Excel, PowerPoint, Canva, or Adobe InDesign to create your poster. Keep it simple (no fancy fonts or excess use of color), and be sure text is easily readable.

Consider turning your podium or poster presentation into an article to further disseminate the information. After all, you have already done much of the work, such as organizing the information. Follow the publication process in Part I, and start work as soon as possible (even before the conference) so you don't lose your momentum.

Write Now!

1. Pick one of the calls for abstracts at https://www.sigmanursing.org/connect-engage/meetings-events/calls-for-abstracts. Download the guidelines and write a submission.
2. Use the guidelines in the chapter and at https://guides.lib.unc.edu/posters/pptwindows2016 to create a poster; the data can be fictitious.
3. List three possible titles for your poster from #2 and describe why you chose the one you did.

    a. ______________________________

    b. ______________________________

    c. ______________________________

4. Visit the website of a professional organization in your specialty area and look for the date of the next conference and when the call for abstracts will be posted. Create a timeline for submitting an abstract for a poster or podium presentation.

CHAPTER 18
From Student Project or Dissertation to Publication

Overview

Academic projects can be turned into published articles, but the work must be transformed to emphasize how it contributes new knowledge and to fit with the targeted publication and its readers. Several steps can help with this process.

Check in with yourself about pursuing publication. Think about your knowledge of the topic: You may have written a great paper but not have the experience with the topic that is needed to write an article. You also want to ask how widely your work can be applied and consider if you are truly committed to the project.

Write a purpose statement. This statement orients the reader to the nature of the article by indicating the aim of the article and how it contributes new or key information related to nursing practice and healthcare.

Determine who will be authors. As noted in Part I, authors must make substantial contributions to the manuscript. A faculty member who provided feedback for your original assignment or advised you on your DNP project doesn't automatically qualify for authorship. Instead, you can acknowledge their assistance.

Decide on the publication venue. Think about which publication would be a good match for your article. Consider publishing your work in multiple areas (making sure that the articles are different from each other). For example, you might publish an article on improving breastfeeding techniques in a nursing journal and in a magazine for the general public.

Choose the article type. When choosing the type, consider the gaps in the current literature, the message you want to convey, and your target readers.

Establish a time frame. Make a plan for the project and stick to it.

Write the article. Create an outline that can guide your writing and incorporate any relevant reporting guidelines. Be sure to format your article according to the publication's author guidelines, including using the correct reference format. Consider graphics such as figures and tables to supplement the text and draw in readers. Once you have completed the article, follow the submission process.

As you write, apply strategies based on the type of academic work. For example, whether you are converting a doctoral dissertation or course-based paper into an article influences how you adapt it for publication. Converting master's research theses and doctoral dissertations requires shortening your work and focusing on what practitioners will want to know.

Transforming your student work into a published article takes time but is worth the effort. You will contribute to the knowledge of others, helping to improve patient care.

Write Now!

1. Choose one assignment that you are passionate about or did well on and research journals and magazines that would be appropriate for an article related to your work.
2. Find out your school's requirements related to sharing work in databases.
3. Create a short outline for a possible article based on a paper you completed for a school project.
4. Download (and use) the School Paper to Manuscript Student Checklist at https://onlinelibrary.wiley.com/pb-assets/assets/17504910/Checklist%20pdfs/6-School-Paper-to-Manuscript-Student-Checklist-1599562514443.pdf.

CHAPTER 19

Writing a Continuing Professional Development Activity

Overview

A nursing continuing professional development (NCPD) or an interprofessional continuing education (IPCE) learning activity tends to be longer and larger in scale, so it can often provide more in-depth information and explore a complicated topic in more detail. You'll want to consider several elements when writing these activities.

Take time to identify a topic that would be of interest to a specific group of practitioners. Look for gaps in knowledge that need to be filled, such as information about a cutting-edge treatment. You'll also want to collect evidence to use as a *needs assessment*, which documents the need for the program. (This assessment is usually required by accrediting bodies.)

An important component of NCPD and IPCE activities are goals and objectives. The *goal* is the purpose of the program, and *objectives* state what behavior is expected of the learner by the end of the program. Depending on the accrediting body, you may be asked to write *outcome statements* rather than objectives. The example below illustrates the difference.

After completing this program, the learner will be able to:

Objective	Outcome Statement
State the four stages of wound healing.	Apply the four stages of wound management to your clinical setting.

Create an outline and be sure to write for your target audience. For example, the amount and type of information about the pharmacological treatment of heart failure will vary slightly between nurse and pharmacist readers. If you are writing for clinicians other than nurses, it's wise to collaborate with someone from that discipline. Keep in mind that interactive teaching-learning strategies such as case studies, exercises, or self-assessment tools enhance learning.

In most cases, you will need to write test questions. Base the questions on the objectives or outcome statements. A common format is the multiple-choice question. As you should throughout your writing project, refer to the author guidelines for test question requirements.

Write Now!

1. State the goal of an educational activity you would like to write.

___

___

___

2. Write two learning objectives related to the goal. For each one, note the level of learning the objective will measure, based on Bloom's taxonomy. The table below may be helpful.

Level of Learning	Type of Learning	Verbs
Knowledge	Memorization and regurgitation	Define, identify, list, repeat, name, relate
Comprehension	Understanding and interpretation	Discuss, describe, report, explain, review, summarize
Application	Use of information in new situation	Translate, apply, interpret, demonstrate
Analysis	Breakup of the whole into parts	Distinguish, compare showing relationships, contrast, differentiate
Synthesis	Combination of elements, forming new structure	Formulate, prepare, design, assemble, plan
Evaluation	Situation assessment, based on criteria	Assess, compute, revise, measure, evaluate

3. Now, instead of objectives, write two outcome statements. Remember to focus on what learners are expected to do after completing the activity. (After completing this program, the learner will be able to…)

4. Pick an NCPD program from a journal and write four post-test questions for it. If you can, compare what you wrote to the published questions.

CHAPTER 20
Writing the Nursing Narrative

Overview

Nurses write narratives for personal reflection, professional advancement, and publication. Types of narratives include advocacy, error, interdisciplinary teamwork, reflection, resilience, and skill acquisition.

When crafting the narrative, describe what you perceived with your senses; share your thoughts, reasoning processes, and feelings. If you're having difficulty writing on the computer (or on paper), try telling your story into your mobile device or a tape recorder, and then transcribe and edit it. Be sure to change any identifying information about the patient.

Narratives can be beneficial for nurses in all types of roles, and writing multiple narratives over time can help with professional growth. Consider a series of narratives over the course of three years from Brian Cyr, MSN, RN, MEDSURG-BC, nursing director of a general medical unit. He reflects on his transition into administrative practice and his practice over time. Reflecting on his three years as nursing director, Cyr writes:

> **2020:** My first year as a nurse director has been intense, challenging, and rewarding. My primary goals were to develop relationships with my staff, assess the strengths and opportunities for development on the unit, navigate the logistical aspects of the role, and develop and utilize my leadership skills. I am grateful for, and appreciative of, the guidance and support of my medical nurse director and physician colleagues, and I am pleased with how I have developed relationships with my staff—it's certainly challenging to get to know over 80 people! Fortunately, my intuitive ability to form good relationships and connect with others that I developed as a staff nurse has served me well. Relating to others and making people feel listened to and valued is one of my strongest skills and one of the aspects of the job I enjoy most. I also have developed strong relationships with colleagues in case management, social work, palliative care, patient advocacy, addiction, and other disciplines that have been very important in navigating some very complicated patient cases this year. This year I developed skills in addressing attendance and professional behavior and filling staffing vacancies. While I'm still developing my approach to these issues, for my level of experience, I'm pleased with the outcomes so far.
>
> Of course, my greatest challenge this year was leading my unit through the COVID-19 pandemic. I wonder if perhaps the pandemic accelerated some of my learnings, and I believe I demonstrated my commitment to my staff to be present and accessible. I am extremely grateful to, and proud of, my entire staff for their dedication, professionalism, and courage in taking on the many challenges asked of them. In addition to my work at the unit level, I continued my role as advisor to the ethics in clinical practice committee and optimum care committee. I also joined two interdisciplinary workgroups—one regarding intrapleural drug administration on general care units and one to enhance staff responsiveness scores across the organization.

Reflecting on year one, Cyr writes:

> When reflecting on this work, it is hard to believe I have only been in this role for one year. In some respects, I still feel quite novice, and yet in other areas I feel much more comfortable and confident. All of this work built upon the early thinking I did preparing for the role, focusing on my vision and values and how they align with the mission of the organization as a whole. As I move into my second year, I look forward to continuing work to capitalize on the strengths of my team in meeting and exceeding the needs and expectations of our patients and families while also cultivating pride, satisfaction, and hopefully joy in their work.
>
> **2021:** It's hard to believe that I have been in the nurse director role for just over two years. Although there are days that I still feel like a novice, reflecting on my accomplishments shows me how much I have developed. Most of my tenure in the role has been during a time of unprecedented change due to COVID-19, which has affected healthcare and especially the nursing profession. In addition, this year we had a successful visit from The Joint Commission. At this point, I have developed solid relationships with my staff and have earned their trust and respect as we continue to navigate these turbulent times in healthcare. I have worked to strike a balance between being transparent and vulnerable while also exhibiting leadership in leading the group in meeting the challenges we face. I am proud of the patient outcomes we are delivering on our unit, and it's clear that the team's efforts are paying off.
>
> This year, I took advantage of many leadership development opportunities, which have been vital in helping me grow and develop as a nurse leader. Building on this work, I served as a mentor for one of two inaugural fellows in the Dorothy Terrell Endowed Diversity Nursing Leadership Fellowship, which helps clinical nurses of color explore potential career opportunities through mentorship. Despite the pressures of the day-to-day work, I try to look for opportunities to support my newer nurse director colleagues or emerging leaders as I have been the beneficiary of mentoring and coaching.

Reflecting on year two, Cyr writes:

> One of the most important lessons I learned from my leadership courses was how critical it is to have a clear and consistent vision and set of values to guide your work and sustain you as a leader, especially in challenging times. While there are many competing priorities in this role, I remain grounded in the vision that a well-educated, supportive, and integrated team of healthcare professionals and support staff working within a strong, professional practice environment can have a profound impact on care delivery.
>
> **2022:** This year I completed my third year in the nurse director role. Though the pandemic has hopefully receded, this remains a very challenging time in healthcare to be a frontline nursing leader. Shifting culture is a slow and steady process, but I see evidence that staff are taking pride in their work, supporting one another, and most importantly maintaining a keen focus on providing high-quality care to our patients and families. Challenges in retaining newer staff persist throughout the industry, and it requires my keen attention on my unit. I have worked with my colleagues in spiritual care and quality and safety to provide

> resiliency rounds to promote well-being. I am also noticing the toll the responsibility I feel toward my staff is taking on me, and I am committed to being more mindful of my own self-care in the coming year. This year I also continued my organizational ethics work, serving as advisor to the ethics in clinical practice committee and fostering the professional growth and development of the two clinician co-chairs while addressing complex ethical challenges clinicians are facing in practice. I participate in the Harvard Ethics Leaders group and serve on the planning committee for the National Nursing Ethics Conference, which has expanded my network of colleagues and resources in the ethics arena.

Reflecting on year three, Cyr writes:

> Expanding my scope to include work external to the organization has been challenging given the pressure of the work to be done on the unit, but it adds value to my role in better understanding the ethical complexity and palpable moral distress facing many frontline clinicians across organizations in our current environment.

Notes on the Narratives

Similar to skill acquisition from novice to expert in any role, Cyr acknowledges how he feels like a novice in his 2020 reflection. During his initial year he primarily focuses on cultivating relationships on his team and with other departments—a process that cannot be fast-tracked but is critical to future success. He also focused on developing skills around personnel management and participated in interprofessional shared decision-making groups. He remarks how starting his leadership role during the advent of COVID-19 may have accelerated his learning. In his 2021 narrative he speaks to how proud he is of his unit's outcomes, which helped contribute to a successful triennial Joint Commission accreditation survey. At the unit level, he was focused on promoting group decision-making and also spoke to his mentorship of nurse fellows interested in administration and supporting newer nurse directors as they transitioned into their new roles. In 2022, Cyr reflected on his work external to the organization as part of a National Nursing Ethics Conference planning committee. Over his three years of reflection through narrative, his leadership skills have evolved, and the scope of his leadership and influence has expanded from the unit to outside the walls of the organization.

Remember: Storytelling is powerful. Depending on the topic, narratives can benefit you, your colleagues, and your patients.

Write Now!

1. Write a narrative. Visualize a patient you cared for or a situation that has stayed with you. Recall what you saw, heard, smelled, and felt. Write the experience as you remember it. Include dialogue and the thoughts and feelings you had at the time. (Be sure to change the patient's name and any other identifying information to protect privacy and confidentiality.) The table below may help you get started.

Information to Include	Your Notes
Name, title, unit, and length of time in practice	
A detailed description of what happened	
Why this situation is important to you	
What your concerns were at the time	
What you were thinking about as it was taking place	
What you were feeling during and after the situation	
What, if anything, stood out to you	

2. Keep a journal for one week to help you identify future ideas for narratives.
3. Use a mobile device or tape recorder to tell a story to yourself, or speak to a trusted colleague about a patient you cared for. Tell it quickly, without judgment or editing yourself. Then listen to the story for key points you might include in a narrative.
4. Review narratives published in *Caring*, a publication of Massachusetts General Hospital, and identify their types.

CHAPTER 21
Think Outside the Journal: Alternative Publication Options

Overview

Alternative publication options, which include letters to the editor, editorials, columns, newsletters, book reviews, and blogs, can help you gain confidence as a writer and provide another way to disseminate key information. These small writing projects may seem more achievable, since many of the options are shorter pieces:

- Letters to the editor are a great way for you to comment on published work, which allows you to suggest solutions to problems, educate readers about an issue, influence opinion, and even bring your work to the notice of others. Be sure to address your "letter," which will be sent via email or an online comments section, to the right person. Start with an attention-getting sentence, be brief, support your point with facts, and end with a call to action or reiterate your main point.
- A guest editorial allows you to offer an opinion and sway readers to share your opinion or take action. Open with a compelling statement, present your position (backed up by facts), acknowledge opposing opinions (and then defuse them), and end with a call to action.
- Columns are short articles for newspapers, newsletters, magazines, or professional journals. (Journals may refer to columns as *departments*.) These are a nice way to get started with writing because they are shorter, and editors need content to fill these since they appear on a regular basis. On the other hand, it can be challenging to "write short," so be sure your topic is focused.
- Newsletters are produced by professional associations, organizations, and institutions. The key is to be sure information you provide is "news" worthy. Like columns, newsletters are an excellent method for getting started in writing for publication because the editors of these have an ongoing need for content. Be sure to have an enticing opening and keep the article short.
- A book review should be more than a description of the book. You want to provide an analysis as to the quality of the book, its significance, and how it relates to practice.
- A professional blog allows you to focus on a specific topic area and provide information on a regular basis. You can start your own blog, but before doing so, be sure you are ready to make a commitment to producing a blog entry on a regular basis (usually at least weekly). An alternative is to contact a current blogger to see if they accept guest blogs.

Many of the basic publishing principles apply with these alternative options: Read the target publication first and follow any guidelines for authors or contributors.

Write Now!

1. Write a letter (email) to the editor and submit it. Read any guidelines before you write.
2. Review your professional association's, school's, or hospital's newsletter. Identify the three main areas that are the focus. What could you contribute as an article in one of these areas?

3. Write a blog on a nursing topic you feel passionate about.
4. Select a journal you read routinely. Does the journal publish columns? If so, read the author guidelines for writing a column. Review the last two years of the journal for relevant and "hot" topics not covered. Contact the editor to see if there is interest in your topic.

CHAPTER 22
Writing a Book or Book Chapter

Overview

A book or book chapter is yet another way for nurses to contribute their expertise. Books in particular require a significant time commitment but can be professionally and personally satisfying once completed.

Think carefully about the purpose of your book, what it would include, who would read it, and how it differs from what is already published. Pitch your idea to a publisher who has released books in line with your idea. As part of the pitch, you'll need to submit a detailed book proposal and provide a sample chapter.

You may choose to fly solo with your book or have one or more coauthors or contributors along for the ride. Each option has pros and cons. Most importantly, if you have a group of contributors, be clear about expectations, and provide detailed information and a template for a chapter (with a sample) to make the contributor's writing process easier and to ensure consistency throughout the book.

As with many writing projects, a key to success in producing a book is to have a detailed timeline to keep yourself on track and meet the publisher's deadline.

Write Now!

1. Compare the table of contents from three different books to identify different formats. Analyze how well the table of contents reflects the book's stated purpose and title.
2. Think of an idea for a book. Using the Sigma Theta Tau International proposal format below, make notes on how you would accomplish each step.

Information	Your Notes
Working title	
Name of the authors, editors, and any contributors already identified	
Description of topic and how the book uniquely addresses a need in the market	
Primary audience	

continues

Information	**Your Notes**
Number of chapters and projected word count	
Special features	
Time frame	
Goals for writing this book	
Competitive works	
Table of contents	

CHAPTER 23
Writing for a General Audience

Overview

You can adapt your knowledge, experience, and scientific writing skills to writing for a general audience, which provides the opportunity to improve society's health. Health literacy, reading level, and cultural and linguistic considerations are key components to keep in mind when crafting your work for the public.

Works for a general audience can take many forms, including articles, letters to the editor, and editorials. In all cases, it's important to know both your target audience and your message:

- Knowing your audience helps you organize and write your content in a way that members of the target audience are most likely to read and potentially act on.
- Knowing your message keeps you focused. You should have only one main message.

Write using plain language to improve readability and understanding. An excellent resource to help with this is www.plainlanguage.gov.

Once you write your article, check for readability through your word-processing program or by using free tools such as the Readability Calculator (https://www.wordcalc.com/readability). You'll also want feedback from those in your target audience.

You can find publishing opportunities by checking magazines found in your local public library and bookstore. Many publications have websites and blogs or are entirely online, offering venues for essays, stories, and practical advice that nurse writers like you can provide.

Write Now!

1. Pick a health-related article on the website of a consumer publication outlet and evaluate it using the checklist for plain language (https://www.plainlanguage.gov/resources/checklists/web-checklist). Rate each item on a 3-point scale, with 3 being completely meeting the criterion.
   - Less is more! Be concise.
   - Break documents into separate topics.
   - Use even shorter paragraphs than on paper.
   - Use short lists and bullets to organize information.
   - Use even more lists than on paper.
   - Use even more headings with less under each heading (questions often make great headings).
   - Present each topic or point separately and use descriptive section headings.
   - Keep the information on each page to no more than two levels.
   - Make liberal use of white space so pages are easy to scan.

- Write (especially page titles) using the same words your readers would use when doing a web search for the info.
- Don't assume your readers have knowledge of the subject or have read related pages on your site. Clearly explain things so each page can stand on its own.
- Never use "click here" as a link. Link language should describe what your reader will get if they click the link.
- Eliminate unnecessary words.

2. Write a paragraph designed for the public, and then test its readability level using the tool in your word-processing program.
3. Pick two or three paragraphs from a published journal article and rewrite them for a general audience.

Before You Go

I hope that this workbook has helped you in your writing journey. Nurses have a professional duty to disseminate their knowledge and expertise—sharing valuable information promotes excellence in practice and improves the lives of our patients. Best wishes for success in your writing endeavors, and remember to follow those author guidelines!

Additional Resources

Here are some resources that may be helpful to you in your writing endeavors.

Tips for Editing Checklist

Here are some questions to ask yourself when editing your article.

Yes	No	
Overall		
☐	☐	Do the title and abstract accurately reflect the content?
☐	☐	Is the tone appropriate for the readership?
☐	☐	Is the text bias-free and respectful to patients (e.g., "patient with diabetes" instead of "diabetic")?
☐	☐	Is the organization of the article logical? Are there any information gaps?
☐	☐	Is the voice consistent? For example, check for switching back and forth from first person (I, we) to third person (he, she, they).
☐	☐	Does the opening make the reader want to read more and set up what is to come?
☐	☐	Are transitions used to move from one point to another and from one paragraph to another?
☐	☐	Are citations and references noted where appropriate but not overused?
☐	☐	Is there a take-home message for the reader? Will the article hold the reader's interest?
Details		
☐	☐	Are the lengths of sentences and paragraphs appropriate?
☐	☐	Have I used active voice when possible and appropriate?
☐	☐	Have I eliminated unnecessary words?
☐	☐	Have I eliminated unnecessary qualifiers such as "might" or "perhaps"?
☐	☐	Are verb tenses (past, present, and future) used correctly, and do subjects agree with verbs?
☐	☐	Do tables, figures, and illustrations support (rather than repeat) the content? Do they have labels, and are they referred to in the text?
☐	☐	Are grammar, punctuation, and spelling correct? Remember to run a final spelling and grammar check.
☐	☐	Are citations and references in the format requested by the publication?

Proofing Checklist

Immediately before submission, do a final proof, checking for the following:

Yes	No	
☐	☐	Are titles and subheads spelled correctly?
☐	☐	Are all organization names spelled correctly?
☐	☐	Are all names of people spelled correctly? Is my biography correct?
☐	☐	Is the sequence of tables, figures, and other graphics correct, and are they called out in the text?
☐	☐	Is each graphic referenced in the text (per author guidelines)?
☐	☐	Are photo and illustration captions accurate, and are people in photos identified correctly?
☐	☐	Are credits for graphics included where needed?
☐	☐	Are tables aligned properly?
☐	☐	Is the math correct in all calculations, and are all numbers correct? (If numbers won't add up to 100%, be sure the reason is stated—e.g., survey results have been rounded.)
☐	☐	Are acronyms spelled out the first time they appear in text?
☐	☐	Are terms consistent? (For example, *healthcare* and *health care* are both acceptable, but pick one and use it consistently. Before picking one, check the publication's style guide for preference.)
☐	☐	If a source is cited within the text, is the complete reference to the work also provided (per style guidelines)?
☐	☐	Are the references formatted correctly, per the publication's guidelines?

If your article is accepted for publication, you may receive a PDF of the layed out article, which shows how it will look when published. If so, be sure to check the above and the following:

Yes	No	
☐	☐	Are pages numbered sequentially?
☐	☐	Is the information in the footer (bottom of page) correct? (The footer typically contains the journal title, volume, and issue date.)
☐	☐	If the reader is referred to another page, is the page number correct?
☐	☐	Are the fonts consistent?
☐	☐	Are headings of different sections the right size, and are sizes consistent? (During the layout process, what should be a subheading may inadvertently be switched to a main head and vice versa.)
☐	☐	Are special characters such as an alpha or beta symbol formatted correctly? (Occasionally these characters don't display correctly.)
☐	☐	Are figure and other captions complete? (Sometimes they can get cut off when imported into the layout program.)
☐	☐	Are online links in the article correct?
☐	☐	Are titles in references italicized per the journal's style? (Sometimes italics are "lost" when going from document to layout.)

If you are proofing a computer-based program, also check the following:

Yes	No	
☐	☐	Can you navigate in the file (e.g., go back a page, return to home, return to the table of contents)?
☐	☐	Are the links active, and do they take you to the correct page?
☐	☐	Do pages contain too much text?
☐	☐	Are all levels of headings consistent in size, color, and font?
☐	☐	Do graphics load onto the page at an acceptable speed?
☐	☐	Can you access help files?

Statistical Abbreviations

You might find this list of common statistical abbreviations helpful in writing and reviewing articles. Refer to the appropriate style guide and author guidelines for information about how to report statistics.

α—Alpha (level of significance, the probability of rejecting the null hypothesis when the null hypothesis is true)

ANCOVA—Analysis of covariance

ANOVA—Analysis of variance

AR—Absolute risk

CI—Confidence interval

df—Degrees of freedom

F—F ratio

f—Frequency

M or $\overline{X}$—Mean

MANCOVA—Multivariate analysis of covariance

MANOVA—Multivariate analysis of variance

Mdn—median

N—Total sample size

n—Subsample size

ns—Not statistically significant

OR—Odds ratio

p—Probability

r—Pearson's correlation

r_s—Spearman rank order correlation

RR—Relative risk

SD—Standard deviation

SE—Standard error

SEM—Standard error of the mean

σ—Sigma, designating the population standard deviation

SS—Sum of squares

T—Wilcoxon signed-rank test value

t—Student's *t* distribution

U or *MWU*—Mann-Whitney U test; also called the Mann-Whitney-Wilcoxon (MWW) test

x^2—Chi-square distributions

References

American Psychological Association. (2020). *Publication manual of the American Psychological Association* (7th ed.). https://doi.org/10.1037/0000165-000

JAMA Network Editors. (2020). *AMA manual of style: A guide for authors and editors* (11th ed.). Oxford University Press.

Tabachnick, B. G., & Fidell, L. S. (2019). *Using multivariate statistics* (7th ed.). Pearson.

Reviewed by Scott Emory Moore, PhD, MSN, RN, AGPCNP-BC, FAAN

Guidelines for Reporting Results

The following guidelines are tools that can help you craft your article. They also help ensure information is presented in a way that facilitates readers' ability to understand your work and evaluate how it fits with their practice. Many of these guidelines, often available in multiple languages, contain a checklist for assessing different sections of the manuscript.

Check the author guidelines to see if a publication requires you to use a specific guideline for reporting your work, and then go to the corresponding website and download what you need. Keep in mind that even if a publication doesn't require you to follow certain guidelines, you can use them to organize and evaluate your manuscript before submission, which may improve your likelihood of acceptance.

If you're not sure which guidelines are best for your project, visit the website for EQUATOR (Enhancing the QUAlity and Transparency Of health Research) Network (http://www.equator-network.org), which includes a searchable database of reporting guidelines as well as a flowchart and online wizard for determining which are the most appropriate for your article. EQUATOR also includes information about additional guidelines not cited here.

The following table is a directory of guideline sources. (Preceding it is a brief bullet list—categorized based on type of study or project—to help you navigate the table.)

- Case reports: CARE
- Clinical practice guidelines: AGREE II, RIGHT
- Economic evaluations of healthcare: CHEERS
- Evidence-based practice: Evidence-Based Practice Dissemination Guide
- Implementation studies: StaRI
- Nonrandomized studies of behavioral and public health interventions: TREND
- Observational studies in epidemiology: STROBE
- Qualitative research: COREQ, eMERGe, ENTREQ, SRQR
- Quality improvement projects: SQUIRE 2.0, SQUIRE-EDU
- Randomized clinical trials: CONSORT
- Reviews: PRISMA

Title	Ideal for Reporting...	Comments
AGREE II (**A**ppraisal of **G**uidelines for **RE**search & **E**valuation) http://www.agreetrust.org/resource-centre/agree-reporting-checklist	Clinical practice guidelines	Checklist available as fillable PDF and Microsoft Word documents
CARE (**CA**se **RE**port Reporting Guidelines) http://www.care-statement.org	Case reports	Website includes a writing template that helps authors follow the guidelines
CHEERS (**C**onsolidated **H**ealth **E**conomic **E**valuation **R**eporting **S**tandards) https://www.ispor.org/heor-resources/good-practices/cheers	Economic evaluations of healthcare	Website includes checklist and video resources
CONSORT (**CON**solidated **S**tandards **O**f **R**eporting **T**rials) http://www.consort-statement.org	Randomized clinical trials	Website includes checklist, flow diagram, and examples
COREQ (**CO**nsolidated criteria for **RE**porting **Q**ualitative research) https://academic.oup.com/intqhc/article/19/6/349/1791966/Consolidated-criteria-for-reporting-qualitative	Qualitative research that includes in-depth interviews and focus groups	Covers three domains: research team and reflexivity, study design, and analysis and findings
eMERGe Guideline https://emergeproject.org/	Meta-ethnography: synthesis of qualitative studies	Website includes video resources
ENTREQ (**En**hancing **T**ransparency in **RE**porting the Synthesis of **Q**ualitative Research) https://bmcmedresmethodol.biomedcentral.com/articles/10.1186/1471-2288-12-181	Synthesis of multiple qualitative studies	Includes 21 items grouped into five domains: introduction, methods and methodology, literature search and selection, appraisal, and synthesis of findings
Evidence-Based Practice Dissemination Guide Dean, J., & Gallagher-Ford, L. (2021) Evidence-based practice: A new dissemination guide. *Worldviews on Evidence-Based Nursing, 18*(1), 4–7. https://doi.org/10.1111/wvn.12489	Evidence-based practice projects	Includes seven steps of evidence-based practice
PRISMA (**P**referred **R**eporting **I**tems for **S**ystematic reviews and **M**eta-**A**nalyses) http://www.prisma-statement.org	Systematic reviews and meta-analyses	Website has checklist and helpful flow diagrams
RIGHT (Essential **R**eporting **I**tems for Practice **G**uidelines in **H**eal**t**hcare) http://www.right-statement.org	Clinical practice guidelines	Website includes extensions, a checklist, and multiple translations

Title	Ideal for Reporting...	Comments
SQUIRE 2.0 (Revised **S**tandards for **QU**ality **I**mprovement **R**eporting **E**xcellence) http://www.squire-statement.org/index.cfm?fuseaction=Page.ViewPage&pageId=471	Quality improvement projects	Website includes examples of well-written items
SQUIRE-EDU (**S**tandards for **QU**ality **I**mprovement **R**eporting **E**xcellence for **E**ducation) https://www.squire-statement.org/index.cfm?fuseaction=Page.ViewPage&pageId=515	Quality improvement projects related to education	Website includes examples of well-written items
SRQR (**S**tandards for **R**eporting **Q**ualitative **R**esearch) https://journals.lww.com/academicmedicine/fulltext/2014/09000/Standards_for_Reporting_Qualitative_Research__A.21.aspx	Qualitative research	Consists of 21 points to address
StaRI (**Sta**ndards for **R**eporting **I**mplementation Studies) https://www.bmj.com/content/356/bmj.i6795	Implementation studies	Includes a 27-item checklist
STROBE (**Str**engthening the **R**eporting of **OB**servational Studies in **E**pidemiology) https://www.strobe-statement.org/index.php?id=strobe-home	Observational (cohort, case-control, and cross-sectional)	Multiple checklists and translations available
TREND (**T**ransparent **R**eporting of **E**valuations with **N**onrandomized **D**esigns) https://www.cdc.gov/trendstatement	Nonrandomized studies of behavioral and public health interventions	Has 22-item checklist

Improving Writing Skills

Bias-free writing—the Conscious Style Guide (https://consciousstyleguide.com) and the Diversity Style Guide (https://www.diversitystyleguide.com)

Grammar Girl website (https://www.quickanddirtytips.com/grammar-girl)—provides grammar advice in an accessible format

Nurse Author & Editor (http://naepub.com)—a free website that contains valuable articles on writing and editing that are written specifically for nurses

On Writing: A Memoir of the Craft (2010), by Stephen King, and *On Writing Well, 30th Anniversary Edition* (2016), by William Zinsser—two classic books on writing

Plain language how-to guide (https://pemsuite.org/How-to-Guides/WG5.pdf)—provides a step-by-step approach for writing plain language summaries

Purdue's Online Writing Lab (https://owl.purdue.edu/owl)—many colleges have writing centers; this is one of the best

Text Recycling Research Project (https://textrecycling.org)—will help you avoid the perils of plagiarism

Writer's Digest (https://www.writersdigest.com/write-better-nonfiction)—has tips for writing nonfiction, most helpful for those writing for a general audience

Style Guides

Here are common style guides. All have online versions that are updated between print publication dates. Most healthcare research and clinical publications use either the *Publication Manual of the American Psychological Association* or the *AMA Manual of Style: A Guide for Authors and Editors.*

American Psychological Association. (2020). *Publication manual of the American Psychological Association* (7th ed.). https://doi.org/10.1037/0000165-000

The Associated Press. (2022). *The Associated Press stylebook: 2022–2024* (56th ed.). Basic Books.

JAMA Network Editors. (2020). *AMA manual of style: A guide for authors and editors* (11th ed.). Oxford University Press.

The University of Chicago Press Editorial Staff. (2017). *Chicago manual of style* (17th ed.). University of Chicago Press.

Search Engine Education

Google Scholar Help (https://scholar.google.com/intl/en/scholar/help.html)—contains tips for finding better results

Medical Subject Headings (MeSH; https://www.nlm.nih.gov/oet/ed/pubmed/mesh/index.html)—free course from the National Library of Medicine

PubMed Online Training (https://learn.nlm.nih.gov/documentation/training-packets/T0042010P)—includes tutorials for both novice and experienced searchers

Publication Outlets

Cumulative Index to Nursing and Allied Health Literature (CINAHL; https://www.ebsco.com/products/research-databases/cinahl-database)—accessed through EBSCO; can download an Excel file or view in HTML a list of journals covered in CINAHL

Directory of Nursing Journals (https://nursingeditors.com/journals-directory)—vetted list from the International Academy of Nurse Editors (INANE) and the publication *Nurse Author & Editor*

Directory of Open Access Journals (https://www.doaj.org/about)—lists open-access journals from around the world; can search by keyword such as "nursing"

EBSCO (https://www.ebsco.com/title-lists)—users can download an Excel file or view in HTML a list of journals for a specific area

National Center for Biotechnology Information (NCBI; https://www.ncbi.nlm.nih.gov/nlmcatalog/journals)—contains journals indexed in the NCBI databases, which includes PubMed; keep in mind that not all quality nursing journals are indexed here

PLOS (http://www.plos.org)—publishes a suite of open-access journals; PLOS Medicine is the most applicable for nurses

ScienceDirect (https://www.sciencedirect.com/browse/journals-and-books)—includes more than 4,700 journals; can search by keyword such as "nursing"

The 2022 "Combatting Predatory Academic Journals and Conferences" report is useful to help you avoid inappropriate outlets (https://www.interacademies.org/publication/predatory-practices-report-English)

How to Conduct a Peer Review

Enhancing the QUAlity and Transparency Of health Research (EQUATOR) Peer Reviewing Research Toolkit (https://www.equator-network.org/toolkits/peer-reviewing-research)

Sense about Science peer review workshops (https://senseaboutscience.org/activities/peer-review-the-nuts-and-bolts-2)

Web of Science Academy Introduction to Peer Review (https://clarivate.com/web-of-science-academy)

Online tutorials from journals and publishers, such as those from Elsevier (https://researcheracademy.elsevier.com/navigating-peer-review/certified-peer-reviewer-course) and Wiley (https://authorservices.wiley.com/Reviewers/journal-reviewers/becoming-a-reviewer.html/peer-review-training.html)

Publishing Guidelines

These organizations publish guidelines for publishers, editors, authors, and reviewers. Author guidelines often state that the publication follows guidelines from one or more of these organizations, with ICMJE the most common.

Committee on Publication Ethics (COPE; https://publicationethics.org/guidance/Guidelines)

International Committee of Medical Journal Editors (ICMJE; https://www.icmje.org)

International Society for Medical Publication Professionals (ISMPP; https://www.ismpp.org)

You can access guidelines for writing different kinds of articles at the EQUATOR Network's (Enhancing the QUAlity and Transparency Of health Research) website (https://www.equator-network.org)

Tools for Creating Better Graphics

You may need a subscription to access a wider range of services, but often the free level provides sufficient help.

Canva (https://www.canva.com)—a web-based graphical design tool

Easelly (https://easel.ly)—guides you through the steps of visually conveying highlights of your work

Mind the Graph (https://mindthegraph.com)—helpful for graphical abstracts and infographics

Piktochart (https://piktochart.com)—includes infographic templates and tips

Venngage (https://venngage.com)—easy-to-use steps help create informative and well-designed graphics

Resources for creating a poster:

- Simplified Science Publishing (https://www.simplifiedsciencepublishing.com/product/free-research-poster-templates)—free poster templates (also search online)
- UCLA Library (https://guides.library.ucla.edu/c.php?g=223540&p=1480858#s-lg-box-4484263)
- University of North Carolina (https://gradschool.unc.edu/academics/resources/postertips.html)

Promoting Your Work

Many publishers have helpful resources.

Elsevier Author Tools & Resources (https://beta.elsevier.com/researcher/author/tools-and-resources?trial=true#3-promotion)

Lippincott: Author Resources (https://www.wolterskluwer.com/en/solutions/lippincott-journals/author-resources)

Springer Nature: Maximize Your Visibility (https://www.springernature.com/gp/researchers/publication-promotion)

Taylor & Francis Group: Research Impact (https://authorservices.taylorandfrancis.com/resources/research-impact-ebook)

Wiley: Author Provided Video Abstract Guidelines (https://authorservices.wiley.com/author-resources/Journal-Authors/Promotion/author-provided-video-abstracts.html)

www.ingramcontent.com/pod-product-compliance
Lightning Source LLC
LaVergne TN
LVHW081253100826
845148LV00009B/1215
9781646481682